COUNTDOWN
TO HEALTHFUL EATING!

Let Corinne T. Netzer be your guide through the calorie maze as you prepare dinner for your family, dine out at your favorite restaurant, or indulge in your favorite dessert. It's easy to plan a sensible food program that includes eating out, snacks, and treats and still stay within your optimum calorie count—with the most authoritative pocket-size calorie counter you can buy!

Updated and revised every year with the newest foods, fresh and packaged, *The Corinne T. Netzer 1998 Calorie Counter* is the perfect reference to help you take the guesswork out of meal planning, make informed, healthful food choices, and take control of your eating.

**THE
CORINNE T. NETZER
1998
CALORIE COUNTER**

D0051892

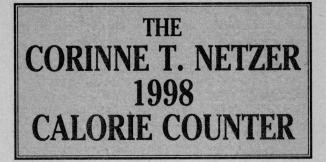

THE
CORINNE T. NETZER
1998
CALORIE COUNTER

Corinne T. Netzer

A Dell Book

Published by
Dell Publishing
a division of
Bantam Doubleday Dell Publishing Group, Inc.
1540 Broadway
New York, New York 10036

ISBN: 0-440-22415-2

Printed in the United States of America

Published simultaneously in Canada

February 1998

10 9 8 7 6 5 4 3 2 1

OPM

Introduction

The Corinne T. Netzer Calorie Counter has been compiled with a twofold purpose: as an annual to keep you up-to-date with many of the changes made by the food industry, and to provide a slim, handy, put-in-purse-or-pocket volume.

My books *The Complete Book of Food Counts* and *The Brand-Name Calorie Counter* are much larger in size and scope, and are therefore much less portable. However, *THIS BOOK CONTAINS MORE PRODUCTS THAN ANY OTHER BOOK OF ITS SIZE!*

To keep this book concise yet comprehensive, I have grouped together listings of the same manufacturer whenever possible. Several brand-name yogurts, for example, are listed as "all flavors." Therefore, instead of three pages filled with individual flavors of yogurt, all with identical calorie counts, I have been able to use the extra space for many other products. And for many basic foods and beverages (such as butter, oil, milk, and alcoholic beverages), I have used generic listings, rather than including the numerous brands with the same or similar caloric values.

Finally, in the process of updating this edition, it was necessary to eliminate many previous listings and brands to accommodate new products and different brands. If you do not find a specific brand-name food that was listed in a previous edition of this book, *this does not necessarily mean that the food product is no longer available.* Also, since food producers are constantly revising and improving products, the caloric counts of your favorite food may have changed even if the description of the product hasn't. Be sure to check for updated entries.

This book contains data from individual producers and

manufacturers and from the United States government. It contains the most current information available as we go to press.

Good luck—and good eating.

C.T.N.

Abbreviations

approx. . . . . approximately
cont. . . . . container
diam. . . . . diameter
fl. . . . . fluid
lb. . . . . pound(s)
oz. . . . . ounce(s)
pkg. . . . . package
pkt. . . . . packet
tbsp. . . . . tablespoon(s)
tsp. . . . . teaspoon(s)
w/ . . . . with

Symbols

" . . . . inch
< . . . . less than
* . . . . prepared according to basic package
directions

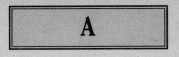

FOOD AND MEASURE   **CALORIES**

A la king sauce mix (*Durkee*), 1 cup* 60
Abalone, meat only, raw, 4 oz. 119
Abruzzese sausage (*Boar's Head Cinghiale*), 1 oz. 100
Acorn squash, baked, cubed, ½ cup 57
Adzuki beans, canned (*Eden* Organic Aduki), ½ cup . . . 110
Alfredo sauce, ¼ cup:
canned (*Five Brothers*) 120
canned, w/mushrooms (*Five Brothers*) 80
refrigerated (*Di Giorno*) 230
refrigerated (*Di Giorno* Reduced Fat) 170
All-purpose seasoning (*Aromat*), ¼ tsp. 0
Allspice (*McCormick*), ¼ tsp. 2
Almond, shelled:
(*Planters*), 1 oz. 170
dried, dry-roasted, or toasted, 1 oz. 167
honey-roasted (*Planters*), 1 oz. 160
slivered (*Paradise/White Swan*), ¼ cup, 1.1 oz. 200
Almond butter, crunchy or creamy, 1 tbsp. 101
Amaranth flour (*Arrowhead Mills*), ¼ cup 110
Anchovies, canned, in olive oil:
flat fillets (*Reese*), 6 pieces 25
rolled fillets, w/capers (*Reese*), 5 pieces 25
Angel-hair pasta:
dry, see "Pasta"
refrigerated (*Contadina*), 1¼ cups 240
refrigerated (*Di Giorno*), 2 oz. 160
Angel-hair pasta entree, frozen (*Lean Cuisine*), 10 oz. . . 260
Angel-hair pasta mix, approx. 1 cup*:
w/herbs or Parmesan (*Pasta Roni*) 320
lemon and butter (*Pasta Roni*) 360
Apple:
fresh (*Dole*), 1 apple 80
fresh, peeled, sliced, ½ cup 32

Apple *(cont.)*
canned, baked (*Seneca*), 1 apple 70
canned, sliced (*Comstock*), ⅓ cup 30
canned, sliced (*Seneca* Sweetened), ½ cup 50
canned, spiced (*Lucky Leaf/Musselman's*), 1.1-oz. ring . . 35
dried, chips, all varieties (*Seneca*), 1 oz. 140
Apple butter, 1 tbsp.:
(*R. W. Knudsen*) 35
spread (*New Morning*) 25
Apple cider, see "Apple juice"
Apple drink (*Lincoln*), 8 fl. oz. 130
Apple drink blends:
berry (*Dole* Burst), 16 fl. oz. 250
cranberry (*Tree Top*), 10 fl. oz. 200
punch (*Minute Maid*), 8 fl. oz. 120
raspberry (*Tree Top*), 10 fl. oz. 190
raspberry-blackberry (*Tropicana Twister*), 8 fl. oz. 130
Apple fritters, frozen (*Mrs. Paul's*), 2 pieces 260
Apple juice, 8 fl. oz.:
(*Apple & Eve*) 110
(*Apple Time/Lincoln/Lucky Leaf/Speas Farm*) 120
(*R. W. Knudsen* Natural/Organic/Gravenstein) 120
(*Mott's* Natural) 120
(*Seneca*) 110
sparkling cider (*Apple Time/Lucky Leaf/Musselman's*) . . 150
frozen* (*R. W. Knudsen*) 120
Apple juice blends, 8 fl. oz., except as noted:
apricot or cherry (*After the Fall*) 100
boysenberry or raspberry (*Heinke's*) 120
cranberry (*Apple & Eve*) 120
grape (*Apple & Eve*), 8.45 fl. oz. 130
orange-banana (*Tree Top* Fiber Rich) 170
pear (*Tree Top/Tree Top* Box) 120
raspberry (*After the Fall*) 90
strawberry (*After the Fall*) 100
Apple syrup (*R. W. Knudsen*), ¼ cup 150
Applesauce, ½ cup:
(*Apple Time* Regular/Granny Smith/Delicious/McIntosh) . . 90
(*Mott's/Mott's* Chunky) 110
(*Mott's* Cinnamon) 120

(*Seneca* Regular/Cinnamon/McIntosh/Golden Delicious) . . 100
unsweetened (*Apple Time/Lincoln*) 50
unsweetened (*Seneca*) 60
unsweetened (*Tree Top*) 70
Applesauce blends:
all blends (*Santa Cruz*), ½ cup 45
w/apricot (*Musselman's Fruit 'N Sauce*), ½ cup 100
w/cherry or peach (*Musselman's Fruit 'N Sauce*), ½ cup . . 90
Apricot, ½ cup, except as noted:
fresh, pitted (*Dole*) 37
canned, in juice (*Libby's* Lite) 60
canned, in heavy syrup (*Del Monte*) 100
sun-dried (*Del Monte*), ⅓ cup, 1.4 oz. 80
Apricot nectar (*S&W*), 8 fl. oz. 140
Arrowroot flour, 1 cup 457
Artichoke, globe (see also "Jerusalem artichoke"):
fresh (*Dole*), 1 medium 60
canned, hearts (*S&W*), 3 pieces 30
frozen, hearts (*Birds Eye*), ½ cup 40
marinated, hearts (*Progresso*), 2 pieces w/liquid 60
Artichoke appetizer (*Progresso*), ⅓ cup 160
Artichoke dip (*Victoria*), 2 tbsp. 30
Arugula, trimmed, ½ cup 2
Asparagus, ½ cup, except as noted:
fresh, boiled, 4 spears, ½" diam. base 14
canned (*Stokely/Stokely* No Salt) 25
canned, all varieties (*Del Monte*) 20
frozen, cuts (*Green Giant Harvest Fresh*), ⅔ cup 25
Atemoya (*Frieda's*), 3.5 oz. 94
Au jus gravy, canned (*Heinz* Homestyle), ¼ cup 15
Avocado (*Dole*), ⅕ medium, 1.1 oz. 20
Avocado dip (*Kraft*), 2 tbsp. 60

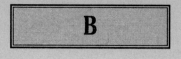

B

FOOD AND MEASURE   **CALORIES**

Baba ghanouj (*Cedar's*), 2 tbsp. 50
Bacon, cooked, 2 slices, except as noted:
(*Black Label/Black Label* Low Salt) 80
(*Jones Dairy Farm*) 90
(*Jones Dairy Farm* Thick), 1 slice 70
(*Old Smokehouse*) 80
(*Oscar Mayer/Oscar Mayer* Lower Sodium/Center Cut) . . . 60
(*Patrick Cudahy*) 80
turkey, see "Turkey bacon"
Bacon, Canadian:
(*Hormel*), 2 oz. 70
(*Jones Dairy Farm Lean Choice*), 3 slices 70
"Bacon," vegetarian (*Worthington Stripples*), 2 strips . . 60
Bacon bits:
(*Hormel*), 1 tbsp. 30
imitation (*McCormick*) 1½ tbsp. 30
Bacon dip, 2 tbsp.:
horseradish (*Kraft* Premium) 50
onion (*Kraft* Premium) 60
Bagel, 1 piece:
plain, onion, or multigrain (*Thomas'*) 150
cinnamon raisin or egg (*Thomas'*) 160
Bagel, frozen, 1 piece, except as noted:
plain (*Lender's* Bagelettes), 2 pieces 140
plain or onion (*Lender's Big'N Crusty*) 220
plain, egg, or onion (*Lender's*) 160
blueberry or cinnamon raisin (*Lender's*) 200
cinnamon raisin (*Lender's Big'N Crusty*) 240
egg (*Lender's Big'N Crusty*) 230
garlic, poppy, sesame, pumpernickel, or rye (*Lender's*) . . 150
oat bran (*Lender's*) 190
soft (*Lender's* Original) 210

Bagel chips:
cheese, three (*Pepperidge Farm*), 1 oz. 140
onion and garlic (*Pepperidge Farm*), 1 oz. 110
onion multigrain (*Pepperidge Farm*), 1 oz. 120
Bagel sandwich, see specific listings
Baked beans, 1/2 cup:
(*Allens*) 150
(*Friend's*) 170
(*Grandma Brown's*) 160
(*Heartland* Iron Kettle) 150
(*Van Camp's* Fat Free) 130
(*Van Camp's* Premium) 140
all varieties except bacon–brown sugar, w/pork, and
    yellow-eye (*B&M*) 170
w/bacon (*Grandma Brown's* Saucepan) 150
bacon–brown sugar (*B&M*) 190
barbecue (*Green Giant/Joan of Arc*) 140
brown sugar (*Van Camp's*) 170
and franks, see "Beans and franks"
honey, bacon (*Green Giant/Joan of Arc*) 160
Mexican style, see "Mexican beans"
w/onion (*Green Giant/Joan of Arc*) 150
w/pork (*B&M*) 180
w/pork (*Green Giant/Joan of Arc*) 120
w/pork (*Van Camp's*) 110
vegetarian (*Heinz*) 140
vegetarian (*Van Camp's*) 110
yellow-eye (*B&M*) 180
Baking powder (*Calumet*), 1/4 tsp. 0
Baking soda (*Tone's*), 1 tsp. 0
Bamboo shoots, 1/2 cup:
fresh, raw, slices 21
canned, drained 13
Banana, fresh (*Dole*), 1 medium 120
Banana, baking, see "Plantain"
Banana, manzano (*Frieda's*), 1 oz. 24
Banana, red, 1 medium, 71/4" long 118
Banana drink (*After the Fall* Casablanca), 8 fl. oz. 80
Banana milk drink, low-fat (*Nestlé Quik*), 1 cup 200

Banana nectar, 11.5-fl.-oz. can:
(*Libby's/Kern's*) 190
blend (*Libby's* Quanabana) 210
Banana squash, baked (*Frieda's*), 1 oz. 18
Barbecue sauce, 2 tbsp.:
(*Hunt's* Light) 25
(*Kraft* Char-Grill) 60
(*Kraft* Original) 40
(*Kraft* Original Extra Rich/*Kraft Thick'N Spicy* Original) . . . 50
(*Maull's*) 40
(*Mississippi*) 60
all varieties (*Stubb's Legendary*) 25
Buffalo wing (*Heinz*) 15
Dijon, mild (*Hunt's*) 40
Dijon and honey (*Lawry's*) 60
garlic, hot or salsa style (*Kraft*) 40
hickory or mesquite smoke (*Kraft*) 40
hickory or mesquite smoke (*Kraft Thick'N Spicy*) 50
honey or onion bits (*Kraft*) 50
honey or Kansas City style (*Kraft Thick'N Spicy*) 60
Italian (*Porino's*) 40
Italian seasonings or Kansas City style (*Kraft*) 45
jalapeño or Kansas City style (*Maull's*) 60
mesquite or mild (*Hunt's*) 40
onion bits (*Maull's*) 45
smokey (*Maull's*) 40
sweet (*Maull's* Sweet-N-Mild/Sweet-N-Smokey) 60
sweet and sour (*Lawry's*) 80
teriyaki (*Kraft*) 60
tropical (*World Harbors Maui Mountain*) 50
Barley, pearled, uncooked, except as noted:
dry (*Quaker* Scotch), ¼ cup 170
cooked, 1 cup 193
Barley flakes (*Arrowhead Mills*), ⅓ cup 110
Barley flour (*Arrowhead Mills*), ¼ cup 75
Barley malt syrup (*Eden* Organic), 1 tbsp. 60
Barley pilaf mix* (*Near East*), 1 cup 220
Basil:
fresh, chopped, 2 tbsp. 1
dried (*McCormick*), ¼ tsp. . . . . <1

Baskin Robbins:

ice cream, deluxe, 1 regular scoop, except as noted:

Baby Ruth, Butterfinger, or *Heath Bar*	300
banana nut, *Baseball nut,* or black walnut	260
banana strawberry, cherries jubilee, peach, or vanilla	240
blackberry, Oregon, ½ cup	140
butter pecan or caramel chocolate crunch	290
cheesecake, all varieties, ½ cup	150
cheesecake, strawberry	270
chocolate or chocolate chip	270
chocolate almond or chocolate mousse royale	310
chocolate cake, German, ½ cup	180
chocolate chip cookie dough or cookies 'n cream . . .	300
chocolate chip mint	270
chocolate fudge or triple passion chocolate	290
chocolate raspberry truffle or world class chocolate . .	280
chocolate ribbon or *Chunk A Cherry Burnin' Love* . . .	250
Choc O The Irish	280
Chocoholic's Resolution	150
coconut, jamoca almond fudge, or strawberry shortcake	280
Everyone's Favorite Candy Bar, ½ cup	170
Fudge, Here Comes the, ½ cup	150
fudge brownie or nutty coconut	310
gold medal ribbon or pink bubble gum	270
jamoca, rum raisin, or decorating vanilla	250
Kahlua and chocolate cream, ½ cup	150
lemon custard or Martian mint	260
Mississippi mudd, ½ cup	160
Naughty New Year's Resolution, ½ cup	170
Nutty or Nice or English toffee	290
peanut butter 'n chocolate	330
peanut butter, *Reese's*	310
pecan caramel fudge, ½ cup	150
peppermint or winter wondermint	270
pistachio-almond	300
pralines 'n cream or *Quarterback Crunch*	290
pumpkin pie or very berry strawberry, ½ cup	130
rocky road or S'mores	300

Baskin Robbins, ice cream, deluxe *(cont.)*
vanilla, French 280
white chocolate, winter 280
ice cream, light, ½ cup:
cherry cheesecake or praline dream 110
chocolate caramel nut 120
espresso 'n cream 100
ice cream, fat free, ½ cup:
berry innocent cheesecake 110
caramel banana or jamoca swirl 110
chocolate marshmallow 120
chocolate vanilla twist 100
soft-serve, caramel praline or vanilla 120
ice cream, no sugar added, ½ cup:
all flavors except berries 'n banana 100
berries 'n banana 80
ices, sherbet, and sorbet, 1 regular scoop, except as
    noted:
daiquiri ice 130
mandarin mimosa sorbet, ½ cup 120
Margarita ice, ½ cup 110
The Mask Twist ice or blue raspberry sherbet, ½ cup 120
orange sherbet or rainbow sherbet 160
peachy keen sorbet, ½ cup 100
pink raspberry lemonade sorbet, ½ cup 120
raspberry-cranberry sorbet, Rudolph's red 140
red raspberry sorbet 140
strawberry island delight ice, ½ cup 100
yogurt, frozen (hard-packed), ½ cup:
brownie madness, Maui, low-fat 140
Caramelcopia 130
Have Your Cake low-fat 110
Jumpin' Java Bean nonfat 120
Last Mango in Paradise nonfat 120
Perils of Praline low-fat 130
raspberry cheese Louise low-fat 130
yogurt, frozen, low-fat, all flavors, ½ cup 120
yogurt, frozen, nonfat, ½ cup:
all flavors except black cherry, coconut, piña colada,
    and vanilla 100

black cherry, coconut, or piña colada 110
vanilla 80
yogurt, frozen, nonfat, reduced sugar, ½ cup:
all flavors except chocolate and whata banana 90
chocolate and whata banana 80
cone, 1 piece:
cake cone 25
sugar cone 60
waffle cone, large 120
waffle cone, fresh baked 146
toppings:
butterscotch, 2 oz. 200
chocolate syrup, 2 tbsp. 90
gummy bears, baby, 75 pieces 130
hot fudge, 1 oz. 100
praline caramel or no-sugar-added hot fudge, 1 oz. . . 90
sprinkles, ⅙ oz. 90
strawberry, 1 oz. 60
whipped cream, Rod's, 2 tsp. 30
Bass (see also "Sea bass"), meat only:
freshwater, raw, 4 oz. 129
freshwater, baked, broiled, or microwaved, 4 oz. 166
striped, raw, 4 oz. 110
striped, baked, broiled, or microwaved, 4 oz. 141
Batter, seasoning (*House of Tsang* Cantonese),
4 tbsp. 120
Bay leaf, dried (*McCormick*), 1 leaf . . . . <1
Bean dip, 2 tbsp.:
(*Frito-Lay*) 40
(*Marie's* Fiesta) 140
black bean (*Old El Paso*) 20
jalapeño (*Frito-Lay*) 40
Bean dishes, mix (see also specific bean listings), Italian
(*Knorr* Cup), 1 pkg. 230
Bean entree, frozen, white, Parisian (*Weight Watchers*
International Selections), 9.87 oz. 220
Bean salad, three:
(*Green Giant*), ½ cup 90
(*Hanover*), ⅓ cup 100
(*Seneca*), ⅓ cup 60

Bean sprouts, see "Sprouts"
Beans, see specific listings
Beans, mixed, canned (*Stokely* Chulent), ½ cup 110
Beans, snap or string, see "Green beans"
Beans and franks, 1 cup, except as noted:
(*Hormel*), 7½ oz. 290
(*Libby's Diner*), 7¾ oz. 330
(*Van Camp's Beanee Weenee*) 320
baked (*Van Camp's Beanee Weenee*) 410
barbecue (*Van Camp's Beanee Weenee*) 340
chili (*Van Camp's Beanee Weenee*), 1 can 240
Beans and rice, see "Rice dishes, mix"
Béarnaise sauce mix (*Knorr*), ⅒ pkg. 10
Beechnuts, dried, shelled, 1 oz. 164
Beef, choice grade, meat only, trimmed to ¼″ fat except
    as noted, 4 oz.:
brisket, whole, braised, lean w/fat 437
brisket, whole, braised, lean only 274
chuck, arm pot roast, braised, lean w/fat 395
chuck, arm pot roast, braised, lean only 255
chuck, blade roast, braised, lean w/fat 412
chuck, blade roast, braised, lean only 298
flank steak, trimmed to 0″ fat, broiled, lean only 256
ground, raw, extra lean 265
ground, raw, lean 298
ground, raw, regular 351
ground, broiled, medium, extra lean 290
ground, broiled, medium, lean 308
ground, broiled, medium, regular 328
porterhouse steak, broiled, lean w/fat 346
porterhouse steak, broiled, lean only 247
rib, whole, roasted, lean w/fat 426
rib, whole, roasted, lean only 276
rib, large end (ribs 6–9), roasted, lean w/fat 434
rib, large end (ribs 6–9), roasted, lean only 284
rib, small end (ribs 10–12), broiled, lean w/fat 376
rib, small end (ribs 10–12), broiled, lean only 264
round, bottom, braised, lean w/fat 322
round, bottom, braised, lean only 249
round, eye of, roasted, lean w/fat 273

round, eye of, roasted, lean only 198
round, full cut, broiled, lean w/fat 272
round, full cut, broiled, lean only 217
round, tip, roasted, lean w/fat 280
round, tip, roasted, lean only 213
round, top, broiled, lean w/fat 254
round, top, broiled, lean only 214
shank, crosscuts, braised, lean w/fat 298
shank, crosscuts, braised, lean only 228
short ribs, braised, lean w/fat 534
short ribs, braised, lean only 335
sirloin, top, broiled, lean w/fat 305
sirloin, top, broiled, lean only 229
sirloin, top, fried, lean w/fat 370
sirloin, top, fried, lean only 270
T-bone steak, broiled, lean w/fat 338
T-bone steak, broiled, lean only 243
tenderloin, broiled, lean w/fat 345
tenderloin, broiled, lean only 252
top loin, broiled, lean w/fat 338
top loin, broiled, lean only 243
Beef, corned:
brisket, cooked, 4 oz. 285
canned (*Libby's*), 2 oz. 120
Beef, dried, cured, 1 oz. 47
"Beef," vegetarian:
burger, see " 'Hamburger,' vegetarian"
canned (*Worthington* Savory Slices), 3 slices 150
canned (*Worthington Prime Stakes*), 1 piece 140
canned, stew (*Worthington* Country), 1 cup 210
frozen (*Worthington* Meatless), 3/8″ slice 110
frozen, corned (*Worthington* Slices), 4 slices 140
frozen, smoked (*Worthington* Sliced), 6 slices 120
Beef dinner, frozen:
barbecue, mesquite (*Healthy Choice*), 11 oz. 310
and broccoli, Beijing (*Healthy Choice*), 12 oz. 300
chicken fried steak (*Marie Callender's*), 15 oz. 650
patty, charbroiled (*Freezer Queen Meal*), 9.5 oz. 250
and peppers, Cantonese (*Healthy Choice*), 11.5 oz. 270
pot roast (*Freezer Queen Meal*), 9.2 oz. 170

Beef dinner, frozen *(cont.)*

pot roast, Yankee (*The Budget Gourmet*), 11 oz.	250
pot roast, Yankee (*Healthy Choice*), 11 oz.	280
Salisbury steak (*Freezer Queen Meal*), 9.5 oz.	260
Salisbury steak (*Healthy Choice*), 11.5 oz.	320
Salisbury steak, con queso (*Patio*), 11 oz.	390
Salisbury steak, sirloin (*The Budget Gourmet*), 11 oz.	260
sirloin (*The Budget Gourmet* Special Recipe), 11 oz.	270
sirloin, meatballs and gravy (*The Budget Gourmet*), 11 oz.	240
sirloin, in wine sauce (*The Budget Gourmet*), 11 oz.	220
sliced, gravy and (*Freezer Queen* Meal), 9 oz.	140
steak patty, charbroiled (*Healthy Choice*), 11 oz.	280
Stroganoff (*Healthy Choice*), 11 oz.	310
teriyaki (*The Budget Gourmet*), 11 oz.	320
tips (*Healthy Choice*), 11¼ oz.	260

Beef entree, canned:

chow mein (*La Choy* Bi-Pack), 1 cup	110
goulash (*Hormel*), 7½-oz. can	230
hash, see "Beef hash"	
pepper steak (*La Choy*), ⅕ pkg.	35
roast, w/gravy (*Libby's*), ⅔ cup	140
stew (*Hormel* Micro Cup), 7½ oz.	180
stew (*Libby's Diner*), 7¾ oz.	290
stew (*Nalley*), 7½ oz.	180
stew (*Nalley* Big Chunk), 1 cup	260
stew (*Nalley* Homestyle), 1 cup	210

Beef entree, frozen:

chipped, creamed (*Freezer Queen* Cook-in-Pouch), 4 oz.	100
enchilada, see "Enchilada entree"	
ground, w/rice (*Goya*), 1 pkg.	860
macaroni (*Healthy Choice*), 8.5 oz.	210
noodles w/ (*Freezer Queen* Family), 1 cup, 8.5 oz.	200
Oriental (*The Budget Gourmet* Light), 9 oz.	250
patty, charbroiled, mushroom gravy and (*Freezer Queen* Family), ⅙ of 28-oz. pkg.	190
patty, onion gravy and (*Freezer Queen* Family), ¼ of 28-oz. pkg.	170
and peppers, w/rice (*Freezer Queen* Homestyle), 9 oz.	210

pepper steak (*The Budget Gourmet*), 10 oz. 290
pot roast (*Freezer Queen* Deluxe Family), 1 cup,
    8.5 oz. 190
pot roast (*Freezer Queen* Homestyle), 9 oz. 170
pot roast, w/potatoes (*Lean Cuisine*), 9 oz. 210
potpie, Yankee (*Marie Callender's*), 10 oz. 690
Salisbury steak:
    gravy and (*Freezer Queen* Cook-in-Pouch), 5 oz. . . . 140
    gravy and (*Freezer Queen* Family), 1/6 of
       28-oz. pkg. 140
    and gravy, whipped potatoes (*Freezer Queen*), 9 oz.   330
    grilled (*Weight Watchers*), 8.5 oz. 260
    sirloin (*The Budget Gourmet* Light), 9 oz. 240
    w/macaroni and cheese (*Lean Cuisine*), 9.5 oz. . . . 290
    w/macaroni and cheese (*Stouffer's* Homestyle),
       9⅝ oz. 350
sandwich, see "Beef sandwich"
shredded, w/rice (*Goya*), 1 pkg. 830
sirloin:
    cheddar melt (*The Budget Gourmet*), 9.4 oz. 370
    in herb sauce (*The Budget Gourmet* Light), 9.5 oz. . . 260
    peppercorn (*Lean Cuisine* Cafe Classics), 8¾ oz. . . . 220
    roast supreme (*The Budget Gourmet*), 9 oz. 300
    tips, w/vegetables (*The Budget Gourmet*), 10 oz. . . . 250
sliced, gravy and (*Freezer Queen* Cook-in-Pouch),
    4 oz. 70
sliced, gravy and (*Freezer Queen* Family), 2/3 cup,
    4.9 oz. 80
steak, patty, grilled peppercorn (*Healthy Choice*), 9 oz. . . 220
stew (*Freezer Queen* Family), 1 cup 180
stew, w/rice (*Goya*), 1 pkg. 770
Stroganoff (*The Budget Gourmet* Light), 8.75 oz. 290
Stroganoff, and noodles (*Marie Callender's*), 1 cup 440
Beef entree mix, Stroganoff or teriyaki (*Dinner*
    Sensations), 1 cup* 320
Beef gravy, canned:
(*Franco-American*), 1/4 cup 30
savory (*Heinz* Homestyle), 1/4 cup 25
Beef hash, canned, 1 cup:
(*Broadcast Morning Classics* Original) 240

Beef hash, canned *(cont.)*
corned beef (*Castleberry's*) 430
corned beef (*Nalley*) 490
roast beef (*Mary Kitchen*) 390
sausage flavor (*Broadcast Morning Classics*) 240
Beef hash, refrigerated, corned (*Jones Dairy Farm*),
 2 oz. 120
Beef jerky, see "Sausage stick"
Beef lunch meat (see also "Bologna," etc.), 2 oz.:
corned, cooked (*Hebrew National*) 80
corned, cooked, round (*Hebrew National*) 60
cut (*Boar's Head* Deluxe Low Sodium) 90
roast (*Hormel/Hormel Light & Lean* 97) 60
roast, Cajun (*Boar's Head*) 80
round, all varieties (*Boar's Head*) 90
Beef sandwich, frozen:
barbecue (*Hot Pockets*), 4.5-oz. piece 340
cheddar or fajita (*Hot Pockets*), 4.5-oz. piece 360
cheeseburger (*Micromagic*), 4.2-oz. piece 370
cheeseburger (*White Castle*), 2 pieces, 3.67 oz. 310
cheeseburger, bacon (*Micromagic*), 4-oz. piece 410
hamburger (*White Castle*), 2 pieces, 3.17 oz. 270
steak, cheese (*Deli Stuffs*), 4.5-oz. piece 370
steak, Philly, and cheese (*Croissant Pockets*),
 4.5-oz. piece 370
Beef sauce, see "Steak sauce" and specific listings
Beef seasoning mix (see also specific listings):
ground (*Durkee* Pouch), ¼ pkg. 25
marinade (*Durkee* Pouch), ¹⁄₁₀ pkg. 0
Beef seasoning and coating mix:
pot roast (*McCormick Bag 'n Season*), 1 tbsp. 10
spareribs (*McCormick Bag 'n Season*), 1 tbsp. 30
Beef spread, roast (*Underwood*), ¼ cup 140
Beef stew, see "Beef entree"
Beef stew seasoning:
(*Adolph's Meal Makers*), 1 tbsp. 20
(*Durkee*), ¹⁄₉ pkg. 10
Beer:
regular, 12 fl. oz. 146
light, 12 fl. oz. 100

Beet, ½ cup, except as noted:

fresh, boiled, drained, sliced 38

canned, all varieties, except Harvard and pickled
(*Seneca*) 35

canned, whole, baby (*Green Giant LeSueur*) 35

canned, whole or sliced (*Green Giant*) 35

canned, Harvard (*Green Giant*), ⅓ cup 60

canned, Harvard (*Seneca*) 90

canned, pickled, all varieties (*Seneca*), 2 tbsp. 15

Beet greens:

raw, 1″ pieces, ½ cup 4

boiled, drained, 1″ pieces, ½ cup 20

Berries, mixed, frozen (*Big Valley* Burst O' Berries),
¾ cup 70

Berry drink, 8 fl. oz., except as noted:

(*Capri Sun Yo Yogi Berry*), 6.75 fl. oz. 100

(*Hi-C Boppin'*/*Hi-C Boppin'* Box) 120

punch (*Tropicana*) 130

punch, chilled or frozen* (*Minute Maid*) 120

Berry juice (*Heinke's* Berry Patch), 8 fl. oz. 120

Biscuit:

(*Arnold* Old Fashioned), 2 pieces 130

(*Awrey's* Round), 2-oz. piece 150

Biscuit, refrigerated, 1 piece, except as noted:

(*Grands! Butter Tastin'*) 200

(*Grands! Butter Tastin'* Reduced Fat/*Grands!* Homestyle) 190

plain or buttermilk (*Ovenready*), 3 pieces 150

baking powder or buttermilk (*1869 Brand*) 100

buttermilk, cinnamon raisin (*Grands!*) 200

buttermilk (*Grands!* Reduced Fat) 190

extra fluffy or Southern style (*Grands!*) 200

flaky (*Grands!*) 190

rich, extra (*Grands!*) 220

Biscuit, frozen, garlic/cheese (*Pepperidge Farm*), 1 piece 170

Biscuit mix:

(*Bisquick*), ⅓ cup 170

(*Bisquick* Reduced Fat), ⅓ cup 150

(*Gold Medal* Biscuit Mix), ⅓ cup 170

(*Gold Medal* Biscuit Mix), 2 biscuits* 180

buttermilk (*Gladiola* Biscuit Mix), ⅓ cup 160

Biscuit sandwich, see "Sausage biscuit"

Black bean dishes, mix:

w/fusilli (*Bean Cuisine*), ½ cup* 174

Jamaican, brown rice (*Fantastic* One Pot Meals),

⅜ cup 140

zesty, and penne (*Fantastic* One Pot Meals), ⅜ cup 150

Black bean garlic sauce (*Lee Kum Kee*), 1 tbsp. 25

Black bean mix, instant (*Fantastic Foods*), ½ cup* 160

Black beans:

dried (*Goya*), ¼ cup 70

canned (*Goya*), ½ cup 90

canned (*Green Giant/Joan of Arc*), ½ cup 100

canned (*Old El Paso*), ½ cup 110

turtle soup, dried (*Arrowhead Mills*), ¼ cup 150

Blackberry:

fresh, trimmed, ½ cup 37

canned (*Allens/Wolco*), ⅔ cup 60

canned, in heavy syrup (*Comstock*), ½ cup 110

frozen (*Stilwell*), 1 cup 100

Blackberry syrup (*Knott's Berry Farm*), 2 tbsp. 120

Black-eyed peas, ½ cup:

fresh, see "Cowpeas"

canned, fresh shell (*Green Giant/Joan of Arc*) 90

canned, fresh shell (*Sun-Vista*) 70

canned, fresh shell, w/jalapeño (*Stubb's Harvest*) 120

canned, dry, w/bacon (*Trappey's*) 120

frozen (*Stilwell*) 110

Blood sausage, 1 oz. 107

Bloody Mary mixer:

(*Mr & Mrs T*), 8 fl. oz. 40

rich and spicy (*Mr & Mrs T*), 8 fl. oz. 50

Blueberry:

fresh, ½ cup 41

canned, in heavy syrup (*Comstock*), ½ cup 110

dried (*Sonoma*), ¼ cup 140

frozen (*Cascadian Farm* Organic), 1 cup 50

frozen (*Stilwell*), 1 cup 90

Blueberry juice (*After the Fall*), 8 fl. oz. 90

Blueberry syrup (*Knott's Berry Farm*), 2 tbsp. 120

Bluefish, meat only:

raw, 4 oz. 141

baked, broiled, or microwaved, 4 oz. 180

Bockwurst, raw, 1 oz. 87

Bok choy, see "Cabbage"

Bologna (see also "Ham bologna," etc.):

(*Oscar Mayer/Oscar Mayer* Beef), 1-oz. slice 90

(*Oscar Mayer* Fat Free), 1-oz. slice 20

(*Oscar Mayer* Light/Light Beef), 1-oz. slice 60

(*Oscar Mayer* Wisconsin Ring), 2 oz. 180

beef (*Hebrew National*), 2 oz. 180

beef (*Hebrew National* Lean), 2 oz. 90

beef (*Hebrew National* Reduced Fat), 2 oz. 130

garlic (*Oscar Mayer*), 1.5-oz. slice 130

"Bologna," vegetarian (*Worthington Bolono*), 3 slices . . 80

Bonito, meat only, raw, 4 oz. 146

Boston Market, 1 serving:

entrees:

chicken, half, w/skin 630

chicken, quarter, dark meat, no skin 210

chicken, quarter, dark meat, w/skin 330

chicken, quarter, white meat, no skin or wing 160

chicken, quarter, white meat, w/skin 330

chicken potpie 750

ham, w/cinnamon apples 350

meat loaf, and gravy 390

meat loaf, and tomato sauce 370

turkey breast, skinless 170

sandwiches:

chicken 430

chicken, w/cheese and sauce 760

chicken salad 680

ham 450

ham, w/cheese and sauce 760

ham and turkey club 430

ham and turkey club, w/cheese and sauce 890

meat loaf 690

meat loaf, w/cheese 860

turkey 400

turkey, w/cheese and sauce 710

Boston Market (cont.)

salads:
Caesar, 10 oz. 520
Caesar, w/out dressing, 8 oz. 240
Caesar, 4 oz. 210
Caesar, chicken 670
chicken, chunky 390
coleslaw 280
pasta, Mediterranean 170
tortellini 380

side dishes, soup, and bread:
apples, cinnamon 250
baked beans, BBQ 330
corn, buttered 190
corn bread 200
cranberry relish 370
gravy, chicken, 1 oz. 15
macaroni and cheese 280
potatoes, mashed 180
potatoes, mashed, w/gravy 200
potatoes, new 140
rice pilaf 180
soup, chicken 80
soup, chicken tortilla 220
spinach, creamed 300
squash, butternut 160
stuffing 310
vegetables, steamed 35
zucchini 80

desserts:
brownie 450
chocolate chip cookie 340
oatmeal raisin cookie 320

Bouillon, 1 tsp. or cube, except as noted:
beef or chicken:
(*Borden* Reduced Sodium) 5
(*MBT/Wyler's* Instant/Low Sodium), 1 pkt. 15
(*Weight Watchers* Instant), 1 pkt. 10
(*Wyler's/Steero/Steero* Reduced Sodium) 5
fish (*Knorr*), ½ cube 10

onion (*MBT* Instant), 1 pkt. 15
vegetable (*MBT* Instant), 1 pkt. 10
vegetable (*Wyler's*) 5
Bow-tie pasta dishes, mix:
and beans w/herb sauce (*Knorr*), ⅔ cup 260
Italian cheese (*Lipton* Pasta & Sauce), ½ pkg. 230
Bow-tie pasta entree, frozen:
and chicken (*Lean Cuisine* Cafe Classics), 9.5 oz. 270
mushrooms Marsala (*Weight Watchers* International
    Selections), 9.65 oz. 280
Boysenberry, ½ cup:
canned, in heavy syrup (*Comstock*) 120
frozen, unsweetened 33
Boysenberry drink (*Farmer's Market*), 8 fl. oz. 120
Boysenberry syrup (*Knott's Berry Farm*), 2 tbsp. 120
Bran, see "Cereal" and specific grains
Bratwurst (*Boar's Head*), 4 oz. 300
Braunschweiger, 2 oz., except as noted:
chub (*Jones Dairy Farm* Original/Bacon/Onion) 150
chunk (*Jones Dairy Farm*) 180
light (*Boar's Head*) 120
light (*Jones Dairy Farm* Chub/Chunk) 100
sliced (*Jones Dairy Farm*), 1.2-oz. slice 110
spread (*Oscar Mayer*) 190
Brazil nut, shelled, 1 oz., 6 large or 8 medium kernels . . 186
Bread, 1 slice, except as noted:
(*Arnold/Arnold Bran'nola* Country) 90
(*Brownberry Bran'nola* Original) 90
(*Merita* Autumn Grain) 80
apple honey wheat (*Brownberry*) 60
apple walnut (*Pepperidge Farm*) 80
bran, honey (*Pepperidge Farm*) 90
bran, light (*August Bros.*), 2 slices 80
bran, whole (*Brownberry*) 60
buttermilk (*Arnold*) 100
cinnamon (*Pepperidge Farm*) 80
cranberry (*Arnold*) 70
date nut (*Thomas'*), 1 oz. 80
French (*Pepperidge Farm* Sliced), ⅑ loaf 120
French, twin (*Brownberry Francisco Intl.*) 80

Bread *(cont.)*

golden, light (*Brownberry Bakery*), 2 slices 80
golden, swirl (*Pepperidge Farm* Vermont Maple) 90
Italian (*Arnold Savoni's*) 60
Italian (*Wonder* 20 oz.) 80
Italian, light (*Wonder* 1 lb.) 40
Italian, thick (*Brownberry Francisco Intl.*), 2 slices 110
kamut, sprout (*Shiloh Farms* Egyptian) 90
mixed grain/multigrain:
   (*Brownberry* Hearth) 90
   (*Roman Meal* Round Top/Sun) 70
   5, sprouted (*Shiloh Farms/Shiloh Farms* No Salt) 90
   7 or 12 (*Roman Meal*) 70
   7, hearty (*Pepperidge Farm*) 100
   7, light (*Pepperidge Farm*), 3 slices 140
   7, light (*Roman Meal*), 2 slices 80
   7, sprouted (*Breads for Life/Shiloh Farms*) 90
   7, white (*Arnold/Brownberry Bran'nola*) 90
   9 (*Pepperidge Farm*) 90
   12 (*Arnold Bran'nola*) 90
   12 (*Brownberry*), 2 slices 110
   crunchy (*Pepperidge Farm*) 90
   nutty (*Arnold Bran'nola/Brownberry Bran'nola*) 90
   w/oat bran (*Roman Meal*) 70
   sprouted (*Shiloh Farms* Sandwich) 80
   whole (*Pepperidge Farm* 100%) 90
nut (*Brownberry* Natural Health) 70
oat (*Brownberry Bran'nola*) 90
oat (*Roman Meal*) 70
oat, crunchy, hearty (*Pepperidge Farm*) 100
oat bran, honey or honey nut (*Roman Meal*) 70
oat bran, light (*Roman Meal*), 2 slices 80
oatmeal (*Brownberry* Natural) 70
oatmeal (*Pepperidge Farm*) 80
oatmeal, light (*Arnold/Brownberry Bakery*), 2 slices 80
oatmeal, light (*Pepperidge Farm*), 3 slices 140
oatmeal, soft or thin (*Pepperidge Farm*) 60
orange raisin or soft oatmeal (*Brownberry*) 70
pita or pocket, 1 piece:
   (*Pepperidge Farm*) 150

(*Pepperidge Farm* Mini), 1 oz. 70
(*Thomas' Sahara*), 2 oz. 150
(*Thomas' Sahara*), 3 oz. 220
(*Thomas' Sahara* Mini), 1 oz. 70
oat bran (*Thomas' Sahara*) 130
onion (*Thomas' Sahara*) 140
salsa (*Thomas' Sahara*) 170
sourdough (*Thomas' Sahara*) 150
wheat (*Thomas' Sahara*), 2 oz. 130
wheat (*Thomas' Sahara* Mini), 1 oz. 60
poppy seed, hazelnut (*Roman Meal*) 110
potato, country (*Wonder* 20 oz.) 80
pumpernickel (*Arnold/August Bros.* 1 lb./*Arnold Levy's*) . . .80
pumpernickel, dark (*Pepperidge Farm*) 80
pumpernickel or rye, party (*Pepperidge Farm*), 8 slices . . 110
raisin (*Arnold Sunmaid*) 70
raisin cinnamon (*Pepperidge Farm*) 80
raisin walnut (*Brownberry*) 80
raisin whole wheat (*Shiloh Farms*), 2 slices 140
rye (*Arnold* Deli) .80
rye, Dijon (*Arnold* Real Jewish) 80
rye, Dijon, thin (*Pepperidge Farm*), 2 slices 100
rye, dill (*Brownberry*) 70
rye, hearty or soft (*Beefsteak*) 70
rye, onion (*Pepperidge Farm*) 80
rye, seeded or unseeded (*Arnold/Brownberry* Natural) 70
rye, seeded or unseeded (*Levy's* Real Jewish) 70
rye, seeded or unseeded (*Pepperidge Farm*) 80
rye, soft (*Arnold* Country) 70
rye, soft, light (*Arnold/Brownberry Bakery*), 2 slices 80
rye, soft, seeded or unseeded (*Arnold Bakery*) 80
rye, thin (*Arnold Levy's Melba*), 2 slices 90
rye and pump (*Arnold August Bros.*) 90
sourdough (*Arnold August Bros.*) 110
sourdough, light (*Arnold*), 2 slices 80
sourdough, light (*Pepperidge Farm*), 3 slices 130
sourdough, thick (*Brownberry Francisco Intl.*) 90
sourdough, whole grain (*Roman Meal*) 70
spelt (*Shiloh Farms*) 100
stick, sliced (*Arnold August Bros.*), 2 slices 110

Bread *(cont.)*

stick, sliced (*Brownberry Francisco*) 100
toast, Texas (*Arnold August Bros.*) 150
Vienna, light (*Pepperidge Farm*), 3 slices 130
Vienna, thick (*Pepperidge Farm*) 70
wheat (*Arnold* Brick Oven) 80
wheat (*Arnold Sunny Valley*), 2 slices 100
wheat (*Arnold/Brownberry* Country/*Brownberry* Hearth) . . 90
wheat (*Brownberry* Natural) 80
wheat (*Home Pride*) 70
wheat (*Pepperidge Farm/Pepperidge Farm* Natural) 90
wheat (*Roman Meal* Natural) 90
wheat (*Shiloh Farms* Homestyle), ½″ slice, 2 oz. 160
wheat, cracked, thin (*Pepperidge Farm*) 70
wheat, dark or hearty (*Arnold/Brownberry Bran'nola*) 90
wheat, light (*Pepperidge Farm*), 3 slices 130
wheat, light or hearty light (*Roman Meal*), 2 slices 80
wheat, light, golden (*Arnold*), 2 slices 80
wheat, sesame, hearty (*Pepperidge Farm*) 100
wheat, soft (*Brownberry*) 80
wheat, very thin (*Pepperidge Farm*), 3 slices 110
wheat, whole (*Arnold* Stoneground 1 lb. 4 oz.) 60
wheat, whole (*Merita* 100%) 70
wheat, whole (*Roman Meal*) 60
wheat, whole (*Wonder* 24 oz.) 80
wheat, whole, light (*Roman Meal*), 2 slices 80
wheat, whole, soft or thin (*Pepperidge Farm*) 60
wheatberry, honey (*Arnold Bran'nola*) 90
wheatberry, honey (*Roman Meal*) 70
wheatberry, honey, light (*Roman Meal*), 2 slices 80
white (*Arnold* Brick Oven) 80
white (*Arnold* Brick Oven 8 oz.), 2 slices 120
white (*Arnold* Country) 100
white (*Arnold Sunny Valley*), 2 slices 100
white (*Brownberry* Country) 90
white (*Home Pride*) 70
white (*Wonder* 12 oz.), 2 slices 100
white (*Wonder* 1 lb.) 60
white, hearty (*Pepperidge Farm/Pepperidge Farm*
    Country) 90

white, light (*Arnold/Brownberry Bakery*), 2 slices 80
white, light (*Roman Meal*), 2 slices 80
white, sandwich (*Pepperidge Farm*), 2 slices 130
white, sandwich (*Roman Meal*), 2 slices 110
white, soft (*Arnold* Country/*Brownberry*) 80
white, soft (*Brownberry* 16 oz.), 2 slices 110
white, toasting (*Pepperidge Farm*) 90
white, thin (*Pepperidge Farm*) 80
white, very thin (*Pepperidge Farm*), 3 slices 110
Bread, brown, canned, plain or raisin (*B&M*), 1/2" slice   130
Bread, frozen, 1/6 loaf:
cheddar, two (*Pepperidge Farm*) 210
garlic or garlic Parmesan (*Pepperidge Farm*) 160
garlic mozzarella (*Pepperidge Farm*) 200
garlic sourdough (*Pepperidge Farm*) 180
Monterey Jack/jalapeño cheese (*Pepperidge Farm*) 200
Bread, ready-to-bake, French (*Pillsbury*), 1/5 loaf 150
Bread, stuffed:
broccoli and cheese (*Stuffed Breads*), 6 oz. 450
pepperoni and cheese (*Stuffed Breads*), 6 oz. 610
Bread crumbs, 1/4 cup or 1 oz.:
all varieties (*Devonsheer/Old London*) 100
garlic and herb, lemon herb, or Parmesan (*Progresso*) . . 100
Italian or plain (*Progresso*) 110
tomato basil (*Progresso*) 120
Bread cubes, see "Stuffing"
Bread mix (see also "Bread mix, sweet"):
beer (*Buckeye*), 1/4 pkg. 130
beer, whole wheat (*Buckeye*), 1/14 pkg. 120
cheddar cheese (*Dromedary*), 1/9 pkg. 140
corn bread (*Ballard*), 1/18 bread* 130
corn bread, buttermilk (*Martha White*), 1/5 bread* 150
corn bread, chili fiesta (*Martha White*), 1/6 bread* 190
corn bread, golden honey (*Martha White*), 1/6 bread* . . . 170
corn bread, Mexican (*Gladiola/Martha White*), 1/6 bread*   130
corn bread, white or yellow (*Gladiola*), 1/6 bread* 140
corn bread, yellow (*Martha White*), 1/5 bread* 140
herb, Italian (*Dromedary*), 1/9 pkg. 140
kamut (*Arrowhead Mills*), 1/3 cup 140
multigrain (*Arrowhead Mills*), 1/3 cup 160

Bread mix *(cont.)*

oatmeal, honey (*Dromedary*), 1/9 pkg. 150
rye (*Arrowhead Mills*), 1/3 cup 160
sourdough (*Buckeye*), 1/14 pkg. 130
sourdough or stone-ground wheat (*Dromedary*), 1/9 pkg. 140
spelt (*Arrowhead Mills*), 1/3 cup 150
wheat, cracked (*Pillsbury* Bread Machine), 1/12 loaf* 130
wheat, whole (*Arrowhead Mills*), 1/3 cup 150
white (*Arrowhead Mills*), 1/3 cup 150
white, country (*Dromedary*), 1/9 pkg. 140
white, crusty (*Pillsbury* Bread Machine), 1/12 loaf* 130

Bread mix, sweet, 1/12 loaf*, except as noted:
(*Buckeye*), 1/16 pkg. 110
apple cinnamon (*Dromedary*), 1/9 pkg. 140
apple cinnamon or blueberry (*Pillsbury*) 180
banana, pumpkin, or nut (*Pillsbury*) 170
carrot or cranberry (*Pillsbury*) 140
cinnamon swirl (*Pillsbury*) 220
date or lemon poppy seed (*Pillsbury*) 180
date nut (*Dromedary*), 1/12 pkg. 180
gingerbread (*Dromedary*), 1/6 pkg. 260
gingerbread (*Pillsbury*), 1/8 loaf* 220

Bread snacks, 9 pieces, except as noted:
crisps, cinnamon raisin swirl (*Pepperidge Farm*), 1 oz. . . 130
crisps, garlic butter swirl (*Pepperidge Farm*), 1 oz. 140
sticks, pretzel (*Pepperidge Farm*) 130
sticks, pumpernickel or sesame (*Pepperidge Farm*) 150
sticks, three cheese (*Pepperidge Farm*) 140

Breadstick:
(*Stella D'Oro* Sodium Free), 1 stick 45
all varieties:
(*Stella D'Oro* Fat Free Original Deli), 5 sticks 60
(*Stella D'Oro* Fat Free Original Grissini), 3 sticks 60
(*Stella D'Oro* Fat Free Traditional), 2 sticks 70
except sesame (*Stella D'Oro*), 1 stick 40
butter or dill and onion (*Awrey's*), 2 sticks 130
cheddar or onion (*Pepperidge Farm* Thin), 7 sticks 70
cheese, three (*Pepperidge Farm*), 9 sticks 140
w/cheese (*Handi-Snacks*), 1 stick 130
garlic and pepper or Italian spice (*Awrey's*), 2 sticks . . . 140

pumpernickel (*Pepperidge Farm*), 9 sticks 150
sesame (*Pepperidge Farm*), 9 sticks 160
sesame (*Stella D'Oro*), 1 stick 50

Breadstick, refrigerated:
(*Pepperidge Farm* Brown and Serve), 1 stick 150
(*Pillsbury*), 1 stick 110
corn-bread twist (*Pillsbury*), 1 stick 140
sesame, thin (*Pepperidge Farm*), 7 sticks 60

Broad beans, fresh, boiled, drained, 4 oz. 64

Broad beans, mature:
dry (*Frieda's* Fava Beans), 1 oz. 15
dry, boiled, ½ cup 93
canned (*Progresso* Fava Beans), ½ cup 110

Broccoli:
fresh, raw (*Dole*), 1 medium stalk, 5.3 oz. 45
frozen, chopped (*Birds Eye*), ⅓ cup 25
frozen, cuts (*Birds Eye*), ½ cup 25
frozen, florets, spears, or baby spears (*Birds Eye*), 3 oz. . . 25
frozen, spears, butter sauce (*Green Giant*), 4 oz. 50
frozen, cheese sauce (*Freezer Queen*), ⅔ cup 50
frozen, cheese sauce (*Green Giant*), ⅔ cup 70

Broccoli combinations, frozen:
and carrots:
  cauliflower (*Green Giant American Mixtures*), ¾ cup . . 25
  water chestnuts (*Birds Eye*), ½ cup 30
  water chestnuts (*Green Giant American Mixtures*),
    ¾ cup 30
and cauliflower:
  (*Birds Eye*), ½ cup 20
  carrots (*Birds Eye*), ½ cup 25
  carrots, cheese sauce (*Green Giant*), ⅔ cup 80
  carrots, corn, peas, butter sauce (*Green Giant*),
    ¾ cup 60
  red peppers (*Birds Eye*), ½ cup 20
  peas, peppers (*Green Giant American Mixtures*),
    ¾ cup 30
and corn and red peppers (*Birds Eye*), ½ cup 50
and green beans, onions, red peppers (*Birds Eye*),
  ½ cup 25

Broccoli combinations *(cont.)*
and pasta, cauliflower, carrots, cheese sauce (*Freezer
   Queen* Family Side Dish), ⅔ cup 70
and red peppers, onions, mushrooms (*Birds Eye*), ½ cup   25
stir-fry (*Birds Eye*), 1 cup 30
Broccoli potpie, w/cheddar, frozen (*Amy's*), 7.5 oz.   . . . 430
Broccoli-cheddar pocket, frozen (*Ken & Robert's Veggie
   Pockets*), 1 piece 250
Broccoli-cheese in pastry (*Pepperidge Farm*), 1 piece . . 240
Broiling sauce, see "Grilling sauce" and specific listings
Broth, see "Bouillon" and "Soup"
Broth concentrate, 2 tsp.:
beef or vegetable flavor (*Knorr*) 15
chicken flavor (*Knorr*) 5
Brown gravy, ¼ cup:
savory (*Heinz*) 25
mix* (*Knorr* Classic) 20
mix* (*Pillsbury*) 10
Brown gravy sauce (*La Choy*), ¼ cup 275
Brownie, 1 piece, except as noted:
(*Hostess* Light), 1.4-oz. piece 140
(*Oreo*) 160
chocolate (*Little Debbie* Low Fat) 190
fudge (*Entenmann's* Fat Free), ¹⁄₁₀ strip 110
fudge (*Little Debbie*) 310
fudge (*SnackWell's*) 130
fudge nut (*Drake's* Reduced Fat) 170
fudge walnut (*Tastykake*) 370
mini (*Hostess Bites*), 5 pieces 260
Brownie, frozen, 1 piece:
à la mode (*Weight Watchers*) 190
frosted (*Weight Watchers*) 100
peanut butter fudge (*Weight Watchers*) 110
Brownie mix, 1 piece*:
(*Betty Crocker*) 180
(*Sweet Rewards* Reduced Fat) 150
blonde, w/white chocolate chunks (*Duncan Hines*) 170
caramel or chocolate chunk (*Betty Crocker*) 190
cheesecake swirl (*Pillsbury* Thick 'n Fudgy) 170
chocolate, dark, w/*Hershey's* syrup (*Betty Crocker*) 190

chocolate chip or German chocolate (*Betty Crocker*) . . . 220
cookies and cream (*Betty Crocker*) 200
dark 'n chunky, chewy fudge, or Mississippi mud
  (*Duncan Hines*) 160
devil's food (*SnackWell's*) 140
frosted (*Betty Crocker*) 210
fudge, dark chocolate fudge, or hot fudge (*Betty Crocker*) 190
fudge (*Betty Crocker* Light) 130
fudge (*Martha White* Moist 'n Fudgy) 150
fudge (*Robin Hood/Gold Medal* Pouch) 170
fudge (*SnackWell's*) 150
fudge, dark or double fudge (*Duncan Hines*) 170
milk chocolate chunk (*Duncan Hines*) 170
peanut butter candies w/*Reese's* Pieces (*Betty
  Crocker*) 200
raspberry dark chocolate (*Duncan Hines*) 150
walnut (*Betty Crocker*) 200
walnut (*Duncan Hines*) 170
white chocolate swirl (*Betty Crocker*) 210
Browning sauce (*Gravy Master*), ¼ tsp. 10
Brussels sprouts:
fresh (*Dole*), 1 cup 40
frozen (*Birds Eye*), 11 sprouts 35
frozen, w/cauliflower and carrots (*Birds Eye*), ½ cup . . . 30
Buckwheat, whole grain, 1 oz. 97
Buckwheat flour, 1 cup 402
Buckwheat groats:
brown (*Arrowhead Mills*), ¼ cup 140
roasted, dry, 1 oz. 98
roasted, cooked, 1 cup 182
Bulgur (see also "Tabouli"):
dry, 1 cup 479
cooked, 1 cup 152
Bulgur pilaf mix (*Casbah*), 1 oz. 100
Bun, see "Roll"
Bun, sweet (see also "Danish"), 1 piece:
apple (*Entenmann's* Fat Free) 150
cheese, blueberry, or pineapple (*Entenmann's* Fat Free) 140
cheese, raspberry (*Entenmann's* Fat Free) 160
cinnamon (*Entenmann's*) 220

Bun, sweet *(cont.)*

cinnamon raisin (*Entenmann's* Fat Free) 160
cinnamon roll (*Awrey's* Homestyle) 270
cinnamon roll (*Weight Watchers*) 200
honey:
    (*Aunt Fanny's*), 3 oz. 360
    (*Aunt Fanny's*), 4 oz. 500
    filled, all varieties except applesauce (*Aunt Fanny's*) . . 350
    filled, applesauce (*Aunt Fanny's*) 330
    glazed (*Entenmann's* Donut Dippers) 160
    glazed (*Hostess*) 320
    iced (*Aunt Fanny's*) 350
pecan roll (*Little Debbie Spinwheels*) 220

Bun, sweet, frozen or refrigerated, 1 piece:

apple cinnamon, iced (*Pillsbury*) 150
caramel (*Pillsbury*) 170
cinnamon (*Pepperidge Farm*) 250
cinnamon (*Sara Lee* Deluxe) 320
cinnamon, iced (*Pillsbury*) 150
cinnamon raisin, iced (*Pillsbury*) 170
orange, iced (*Pillsbury*) 170

Burbot, meat only, baked, broiled, or microwaved,
    4 oz. 130

Burger King, 1 serving:

breakfast:
    biscuit w/bacon, egg, and cheese 510
    biscuit w/sausage 590
    Croissan'wich, sausage, egg, and cheese 600
    French toast sticks 500
    hash browns 220
    A.M. Express jam, grape or strawberry 30
sandwiches:
    BK Big Fish 700
    BK Broiler chicken 550
    cheeseburger, regular 380
    cheeseburger, double 600
    cheeseburger, double, w/bacon 640
    chicken sandwich 710
    Double Whopper 870
    Double Whopper w/cheese 960

hamburger 330
Whopper 640
Whopper w/cheese 730
Whopper Jr. 420
Whopper Jr. w/cheese 460
Chicken Tenders, 8 pieces 310
dipping sauces, 1 oz., except as noted:
   A.M. Express 80
   barbecue 35
   Bull's Eye, 1/2 oz. 40
   honey 90
   ranch 170
   sweet and sour 45
side dishes:
   fries, medium 370
   fries, coated, medium 340
   onion rings 310
salad w/out dressing:
   chicken, broiled 200
   garden 100
   side 60
salad dressings, 1.1 oz.:
   bleu cheese 160
   French or Thousand Island 140
   Italian, light 15
   ranch 180
desserts and shakes:
   Dutch apple pie 300
   shake, chocolate, medium 320
   shake, chocolate w/syrup, medium 440
   shake, strawberry w/syrup, medium 420
   shake, vanilla, medium 300
Burrito, frozen, 1 piece or pkg.:
bean, black (*Amy's*), 6 oz. 320
bean and cheese (*Old El Paso*), 5 oz. 300
bean and rice (*Amy's*), 6 oz. 250
bean, rice and cheese (*Amy's*), 6 oz. 280
beef (*Hormel Quick Meal*), 4 oz. 300
beef and bean, all varieties (*Old El Paso*), 5 oz. 320
cheese (*Hormel Quick Meal*), 4 oz. 250

Burrito *(cont.)*

chicken con queso (*Healthy Choice*), 10.55 oz. 360
chili, red (*Hormel Quick Meal*), 4 oz. 280
pizza, cheese (*Old El Paso*), 3.5 oz. 240
pizza, pepperoni (*Old El Paso*), 3.5 oz. 260
pizza, sausage (*Old El Paso*), 3.5 oz. 250
Burrito, breakfast, frozen, black bean (*Amy's*), 1 pkg. . . 230
Burrito mix (*Old El Paso* Dinner), 1 piece* 280
Burrito sauce (*Hunt's Manwich*), ¼ cup 25
Burrito seasoning mix (*Old El Paso*), 2 tsp. 15
Butter (see also "Margarine"):
(*Land O Lakes* Light), 1 tsp. 50
regular, salted or unsalted, 1 tbsp. 100
whipped, 1 tbsp. 67
Butter beans, see "Lima beans"
Butter salt (*Durkee*), ½ tsp. 0
Butterfish, meat only:
raw, 4 oz. 166
baked, broiled, or microwaved, 4 oz. 212
Buttermilk, see "Milk"
Butternut, dried, shelled, 1 oz. 174
Butternut squash:
fresh, baked, cubed, ½ cup 41
frozen, 12-oz. pkg. 192
Butterscotch chips, baking (*Nestlé* Morsels), 1 tbsp. 80
Butterscotch topping, 2 tbsp.:
(*Smucker's* Sundae) 110
caramel (*Smucker's* Nonfat/*Smucker's* Special Recipe) . . 130
or butterscotch caramel fudge (*Mrs. Richardson's*) 130

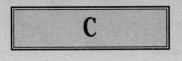

FOOD AND MEASURE   **CALORIES**

Cabbage, ½ cup, except as noted:
fresh, raw, shredded 9
fresh, boiled, drained, shredded 17
bok choy, fresh, raw, shredded 5
bok choy, fresh, boiled, drained, shredded 10
napa, fresh, raw, shredded (*Dole*), 3 oz. 6
pe-tsai, fresh, raw, shredded 6
pe-tsai, fresh, boiled, drained, shredded 8
red, fresh, boiled, drained, shredded 16
red, canned (*Seneca*) 80
red, in jars, sweet and sour (*Greenwood*) 100
savoy, fresh, boiled, drained, shredded 18
Cabbage entree, stuffed, w/potato, frozen (*Lean
    Cuisine*), 9.5 oz. 180
Cactus, marinated (*Goya* Napolitos), 2–3 pieces 20
Caesar salad, see "Salad blend mix"
Cake, frozen:
Boston creme (*Pepperidge Farm*), ⅛ cake 260
carrot (*Pepperidge Farm Deluxe*), ⅛ cake 310
cheesecake:
    (*Sara Lee* Original Cream), ¼ cake 330
    triple chocolate (*Weight Watchers*), 3.15-oz. cake . . . 200
    French (*Sara Lee*), ⅕ cake 410
    French style (*Weight Watchers*), 3.9-oz. cake 180
    New York style (*Weight Watchers*), 2.5-oz. cake 150
    strawberry (*Amy's*), 4 oz. 290
    strawberry, French (*Sara Lee*), ⅙ cake 320
chocolate:
    double, layer (*Sara Lee*), ⅛ cake 260
    fudge or German, layer (*Pepperidge Farm*),
        ⅙ cake 300
    fudge stripe layer (*Pepperidge Farm*), ⅙ cake 290
    mousse (*Pepperidge Farm*), ⅛ cake 250

Cake, frozen, chocolate *(cont.)*
   mousse (*Sara Lee*), 1/5 cake 400
   raspberry royale (*Weight Watchers*), 3.5 oz. 190
coconut or German chocolate (*Sara Lee*), 1/8 cake 280
coffee cake (*Sara Lee*), 1/8 cake 220
coffee cake (*Sara Lee* Reduced Fat), 1/6 cake 180
coffee cake, raspberry (*Sara Lee*), 1/6 cake 200
fudge, double (*Weight Watchers*), 2.75-oz. cake 190
golden layer, fudge (*Sara Lee*), 1/8 cake 270
pound (*Sara Lee* Reduced Fat), 1/4 cake 280
pound, butter (*Sara Lee*), 1/4 cake 320
pound, chocolate swirl (*Sara Lee*), 1/4 cake 330
pound, strawberry swirl (*Sara Lee*), 1/4 cake 290
Cake, snack (see also specific listings):
(*Tastykake Koffee Kake*), 2.5 oz. 270
(*Tastykake Kreme Krimpies*), 2 pieces 230
apple filled (*Tastykake Krimpets* Low Fat), 2 pieces 160
apple raisin (*SnackWell's*), 1 piece 130
banana (*SnackWell's*), 1 piece 130
banana (*Tastykake* Creamies), 1 piece 170
butterscotch iced (*Tastykake Krimpets*), 2 pieces 210
chocolate:
   (*Devil Dogs*), 1.6 oz. 170
   (*Hostess Choco Licious*), 2 pieces 370
   (*Ring Dings*), 2 pieces 320
   (*Tastykake* Creamies), 1 piece 180
   cherry (*SnackWell's*), 1 piece 130
chocolate chip (*Chips Ahoy!*), 1 piece 150
coconut covered (*Tastykake* Juniors), 1 piece 320
coffee cake (*Drake's* Low Fat), 1 piece 100
coffee cake (*Little Debbie*), 1 piece 230
crumb (*Hostess* Light), 3 pieces 260
cupcake, 2 pieces:
   (*Tastykake Kreme Kup*) 190
   (*Yankee Doodles*) 220
   buttercreme, iced (*Tastykake*) 250
   chocolate (*Hostess* Light) 270
   chocolate (*Tastykake*) 220
   chocolate creme (*Tastykake* Low Fat) 200
   creme (*Tastykake Koffee Kake*) 240

filled, all varieties (*Tastykake Koffee Kake* Low Fat) . . 160
vanilla, creme (*Tastykake* Low Fat) 210
golden:
   (*SnackWell's*), 1 piece 130
   creme-filled (*Hostess* Dessert Cup), 1 piece 90
   creme-filled (*Sunny Doodles*), 2 pieces 220
   creme-filled (*Sunny Doodles* Reduced Fat), 2 pieces   180
   creme-filled (*Twinkies*), 1.4 oz. 140
   creme-filled (*Twinkies* Light), 1.4 oz. 120
jelly/lemon filled (*Tastykake Krimpets* Low Fat), 2 pieces 180
peanut butter (*Tastykake Kandy Kakes*), 3 pieces 280
sprinkled (*Tastykake* Creamies), 1 piece 150
stick, dunking (*Tastykake* Stix), 1 piece 190
strawberry, iced (*Tastykake Krimpets*), 2 pieces 210
vanilla (*Tastykake* Creamies), 1 piece 190
Cake, snack, mix*:
(*Betty Crocker* Easy Layer Bar), 1 bar 140
apple cinnamon (*Sweet Rewards*), ⅛ cake 170
apple streusel bar (*Pillsbury*), 1 bar 150
Boston cream pie (*Betty Crocker*), ¹/₁₀ pie 200
caramel oatmeal bar (*Betty Crocker*), 1 bar 180
cheesecake bar, strawberry swirl (*Betty Crocker*),
   1 bar 210
chocolate chip bar (*Pillsbury Chips Ahoy!*), 1 bar 150
chocolate chunk bar (*Betty Crocker*), 1 bar 120
chocolate peanut butter bar (*Betty Crocker*), 1 bar . . . 200
chocolate pudding (*Betty Crocker*), ⅛ cake 170
cookie bar, 1 bar:
   (*Betty Crocker Hershey*) 140
   (*Betty Crocker M&M's*) 170
   (*Pillsbury M&M's*) 170
   chocolate (*Pillsbury Oreo*) 180
   double decker (*Duncan Hines*) 130
   fudge swirl (*Pillsbury*) 180
   milk chocolate chunk (*Duncan Hines*) 140
cupcake, dirt (*Duncan Hines*), 2 pieces 300
cupcake, polka dot angel food (*Duncan Hines*),
   3 pieces 160
date bar (*Betty Crocker*), ¹/₁₂ pkg. 150
gingerbread (*Betty Crocker*), ⅛ pkg. 230

Cake, snack, mix *(cont.)*
lemon (*Sweet Rewards*), ⅛ cake 170
lemon bar (*Betty Crocker Sunkist*), 1 bar 140
lemon cheesecake bar (*Pillsbury*), 1 bar 190
lemon chiffon (*Betty Crocker*), 1/16 cake 140
lemon pudding (*Betty Crocker*), ⅛ cake 180
peanut butter bar (*Pillsbury Nutter Butter*), 1 bar 180
pineapple upside-down cake (*Betty Crocker*), ⅙ cake . . . 400
pound cake (*Betty Crocker*), ⅛ cake 290
raspberry bar (*Betty Crocker*), 1 bar 170
S'mores bar (*Betty Crocker*), 1 bar 180
Cake decoration (see also "Frosting"):
confetti, nonpareils, holiday sprinkles, rainbows, sugar
    crystals, or trims (*Dec-A-Cake*), 1 tsp. 15
sprinkles (*Hershey's* Cookies n' Mint), 2 tbsp. 100
sprinkles, milk chocolate (*Hershey's*), 2 tbsp. 140
Cake mix, 1/12 cake*, except as noted:
angel food (*Duncan Hines*) 140
angel food, lemon custard, or white (*SuperMoist*) 140
angel food, strawberry (*Duncan Hines*) 130
banana (*Duncan Hines* Supreme) 250
butter pecan (*SuperMoist*) 250
butter recipe, chocolate (*SuperMoist*) 270
butter recipe, fudge or golden (*Duncan Hines*),
    1/10 cake* 320
butter recipe, yellow (*SuperMoist*) 260
caramel, wild cherry, or butterscotch (*Duncan Hines*) . . . 250
carrot (*SuperMoist*), 1/10 cake* 300
cheesecake (*Jell-O* Homestyle), ⅙ cake* 360
cheesecake, blueberry (*Jell-O*), ⅙ cake* 320
cheesecake, strawberry (*Jell-O*), ⅙ cake* 340
cherry chip (*SuperMoist*), 1/10 cake* 280
chip, rainbow (*SuperMoist*) 250
chocolate, fudge or milk (*SuperMoist*) 250
chocolate, German (*SuperMoist*) 250
chocolate chip (*SuperMoist*) 280
chocolate swirl, double (*SuperMoist*) 250
devil's food (*Robin Hood* Pouch), ⅕ cake* 310
devil's food (*SnackWell's*), ⅙ cake* 200
devil's food (*SuperMoist*) 240

devil's food (*SuperMoist* Light), 1/10 cake* 230
lemon (*Duncan Hines* Supreme) 250
lemon (*SuperMoist*) 250
lime, key (*Duncan Hines*) 250
marble, fudge (*Duncan Hines*) 250
marble, fudge (*SuperMoist*) 250
pineapple or orange (*Duncan Hines* Supreme) 250
pound (*Betty Crocker*), 1/8 pkg. 270
raspberry or spice (*Duncan Hines*) 250
spice (*SuperMoist*) 250
strawberry (*Duncan Hines* Supreme) 250
strawberry swirl (*SuperMoist*), 1/10 cake* 290
swirl, party (*SuperMoist*) 250
swirl, peanut butter chocolate (*SuperMoist*) 240
swirl, white chocolate (*SuperMoist*) 250
vanilla, French (*Duncan Hines*) 250
vanilla, French (*SuperMoist*) 250
vanilla, golden (*SuperMoist*) 280
white (*Duncan Hines*) 240
white (*SnackWell's*), 1/6 cake* 210
white (*SuperMoist*) 230
white (*SuperMoist* Light), 1/10 cake* 210
white, Olympic party (*SuperMoist*) 240
white, sour cream (*SuperMoist*), 1/10 cake* 280
yellow (*Duncan Hines*) 250
yellow (*SnackWell's*), 1/6 cake* 210
yellow (*SuperMoist*) 240
yellow (*SuperMoist* Light), 1/10 cake* 230
Canary beans, dry (*Goya*), 1/4 cup 190
Candy:
(*Baby Ruth*), 2.1-oz. bar 280
(*Bar None*), 1.65-oz. bar 250
(*Buncha Crunch*), 1.4 oz. 200
all flavors (*Pearson Nips*), 2 pieces 60
buttercrunch, w/almonds (*Almond Roca*), 4 pieces 280
(*Butterfinger*), 2.1-oz. bar 280
(*Butterfinger BB's*), 1.7-oz. bag 230
candy cane (*Starburst*), 1 piece 70
candy corn (*Heide/Heide Indian*), 1 oz. 110
caramel (*Kraft*), 5 pieces 170

Candy *(cont.)*

caramel, chocolate coated (*Milk Duds*), 1.85-oz. box . . . 230
caramel, w/cookies (*Twix* Singles), 2 bars, 2 oz. 280
caramel, and peanut butter (*Hershey's Sweet Escapes*),
   1.4-oz. bar 150
chocolate (*Cella's* Dark/Milk), 2 pieces, 1 oz. 110
chocolate, candy coated:
   (*M&M's*), 1.5 oz. 210
   w/almonds (*M&M's*), 1.5 oz. 230
   mini (*M&M's Tube*), 1¼-oz. tube 170
   peanut butter (*M&M's*), 1.5 oz. 220
   w/peanuts (*M&M's*), 1.5 oz. 220
chocolate, dark:
   (*Dove* Mini), 7 pieces, 1.5 oz. 220
   (*Dove* Singles), 1.3-oz. bar 200
   (*Hershey's Special Dark*), 1.45-oz. bar 230
   bittersweet (*Toblerone*), ⅓ of 3.5-oz. bar 180
chocolate, milk:
   (*Dove* Mini), 7 pieces, 1.5 oz. 230
   (*Dove* Single), 1.3-oz. bar 200
   (*Hershey's*), 1.55-oz. bar 230
   (*Hershey's Hugs*), 8 pieces 200
   (*Hershey's Miniatures*), 5 pieces 230
   (*Nestlé*), 1.45-oz. bar 220
   (*Symphony*), 1.5-oz. bar 230
   plain or w/almonds (*Hershey's Kisses*), 8 pieces . . . 210
   plain or w/almonds (*Hershey's* Nuggets), 4 pieces . . 210
   w/almonds (*Cadbury*), 9 blocks 220
   w/almonds (*Hershey's*), 1.45-oz. bar 230
   w/almonds (*Hershey's* Golden), 2.8-oz. bar 450
   w/almonds (*Hershey's Hugs*), 9 pieces 230
   w/almonds and toffee (*Symphony*), 1.5-oz. bar 240
   cookies and cream (*Hershey's* Nuggets), 4 pieces . . . 200
   w/crisps (*Cadbury* Krisp), 9 blocks 200
   w/crisps (*Crunch*), 1.55-oz. bar 230
   w/crisps (*Krackel*), 1.4-oz. bar 220
   w/honey and nougat (*Toblerone*), ⅓ of 3.5-oz. bar . . 180
   w/macadamias (*Hershey's* Golden), 2.4-oz. bar 380
   w/peanuts (*Mr. Goodbar*), 1¾-oz. bar 270

chocolate, triple, wafer (*Hershey's Sweet Escapes*),
  1.4-oz. bar 160
chocolate toffee crisp (*Hershey's Sweet Escapes*),
  1.4-oz. bar 190
chocolate mint:
  (*Cadbury* Mint), 5 blocks 190
  candy coated (*M&M's*), 1.5 oz. 200
  cookies and (*Hershey's*), 1.55-oz. bar 230
  cookies and (*Hershey's* Nuggets), 4 pieces 200
chocolate, white:
  w/cookie (*Hershey's Cookies 'n' Creme*),
    1.5-oz. bar 230
  w/crisps (*Nestlé White Crunch*), 1.4-oz. bar 220
coconut, chocolate coated (*Mounds*), 1.9-oz. bar 250
coconut, w/almonds, chocolate coated (*Almond Joy*),
  1.76-oz. bar 240
fruit flavor:
  all flavors (*Skittles*), 1.5 oz. 170
  chews, all flavors (*Starburst*), 8 pieces, 1.4 oz. . . 160
  twists (*Starburst*), 4 pieces, 1.5 oz. 140
  gummed, all flavors (*Dots*), 12 pieces, 1.5 oz. 150
fudge (*Kraft* Fudgies), 5 pieces, 1.4 oz. 180
gum, chewing, all flavors (*Care*Free*), 1 piece 10
gum, bubble (*Care*Free*), 1 stick 5
halvah, chocolate (*Joyva*), 1.75 oz. 340
hard, all flavors (*Hershey's Tastetations*), 3 pieces . . . 60
hard, all flavors (*Lifesavers*), 2 pieces 20
hard, all flavors (*Tootsie Pop* Drops) 1 piece, .2 oz. . . . 20
jelled, spearmint leaves (*Brach's*), 5 pieces 130
jelly beans, all flavors (*Jelly Belly*), 35 pieces, 1.4 oz. . . 140
licorice, black or strawberry (*Twizzlers*), 4 pieces . . . 140
licorice, cherry (*Twizzlers*), 4 pieces 150
licorice, chocolate (*Twizzlers*), 5 pieces 140
licorice, candy coated (*Good & Fruity*), 1.8-oz. box . . . 150
lollipop, all flavors (*Charms*), .5-oz. pop 60
malted milk balls (*Whoppers*), 1.4 oz. 190
(*Mars*), 1.76-oz. bar 240
marshmallow, mini (*Kraft*), ½ cup 100
(*Milky Way* Original Singles), 2-oz. bar 270
(*Milky Way* Dark Singles), 1.76-oz. bar 220

Candy *(cont.)*
(*Milky Way* Lite Singles), 1.57-oz. bar 170
mint, butter (*Kraft*), 7 pieces 60
mint, chocolate coated (*Junior* Mints), 16 pieces 160
mint, chocolate coated (*York* Peppermint Pattie),
  1.5-oz. piece 150
(*Nestlé Turtles*), 2 pieces 160
nonpareils (*Sno-Caps*), 2.3 oz. 300
nougat (*Charleston Chew* Vanilla), 5 pieces, 1.2 oz. 150
(*Nutrageous*), 1.6-oz. bar 240
(*Oh Henry!*), 1.8-oz. bar 230
(*100 Grand*), 1.5-oz. bar 200
(*Pay Day*), 1.85-oz. bar 250
peanut, chocolate coated (*Goobers*), 1.38 oz. 210
peanut butter, chocolate (*5th Avenue*), 2-oz. bar 280
peanut butter, w/cookie (*Twix*), .9-oz. bar 130
peanut butter cup (*Reese's*), 2 pieces, 1.6-oz. pkg. 240
peanut butter cup (*Reese's* Crunchy), 2 pieces,
  1.6 oz. 250
popcorn, caramel, see "Popcorn, popped"
raisins, yogurt coated (*Del Monte*), .9-oz. bag 110
(*Snickers* Miniatures), 4 pieces, 1.26 oz. 170
(*Snickers* Singles), 2.07-oz. bar 280
(*Sugar Babies*), 30 pieces 180
(*Sugar Daddy* Chewz), 5 pieces, 1.5 oz. 160
(*3 Musketeers*), 2.13-oz. bar 260
toffee bar (*Heath*), 1.4 oz. 210
(*Tootsie Roll* Midges), 6 pieces, 1.4 oz. 160
(*Whatchamacallit*), 1.7-oz. bar 250
Cannellini beans, see "Kidney beans"
Cannelloni dinner, frozen (*Amy's*), 10 oz. 260
Cannelloni entree, frozen, cheese (*Lean Cuisine*), 9⅛ oz. 230
Cantaloupe (*Dole*), ¼ fruit 50
Capers (*B&G*), 1 tbsp. 5
Caperberries, in jars (*Haddon House*), ½ oz. 0
Carambola, fresh (*Frieda's*), 3.5 oz. 35
Caramel dip (*Marie's* Low Fat), 2 tbsp. 140
Caramel topping, 2 tbsp.:
(*Kraft*) 120
(*Mrs. Richardson's* Fat Free) 130

Caraway seed (*McCormick*), ¼ tsp. 4
Cardoon:
raw, shredded, ½ cup 18
boiled, drained, 4 oz. 25
Carissa, 1 medium, .8 oz. 12
Carob flour, 1 cup 395
Carp, meat only:
raw, 4 oz. 144
baked, broiled, or microwaved, 4 oz. 184
Carrot:
fresh, raw, whole (*Dole*), 7″ long, 2.8 oz. 35
fresh, raw, shredded or peeled mini (*Dole*), 3 oz. 40
canned, all varieties (*Seneca*), ½ cup 25
canned, baby, whole (*LeSueur*), ½ cup 35
canned, sliced (*Green Giant*), ½ cup 25
frozen, baby, whole (*Birds Eye*), ½ cup 40
frozen, sliced (*Birds Eye*), ½ cup 35
Carvel:
ice cream, soft serve, ½ cup:
  chocolate 180
  chocolate, no fat 90
  vanilla 190
  vanilla, no fat 120
sherbet, all flavors, ½ cup 150
yogurt, soft serve, vanilla, no sugar, ½ cup 100
novelties, 1 piece:
  Brown Bonnet cone 380
  Chipsters 380
  Flying Saucer 240
  ice cream cupcake 210
Casaba pulp, cubed, ½ cup 23
Cashew, 1 oz., except as noted:
(*Frito-Lay*), 1.5 oz. 270
whole (*Paradise/White Swan*), ¼ cup, 1.2 oz. 210
dry-roasted or oil-roasted, 1 oz. or 18 medium 163
oil-roasted (*Master Choice*) 170
oil-roasted (*Planters*), 1-oz. pkg. 160
honey-roasted (*Planters*) 150
Cashew butter (*Roaster Fresh*), 1 oz. 165

Catfish, channel, meat only, 4 oz.:

farmed, raw 153
farmed, baked, broiled, or microwaved 172
wild, raw 108
wild, baked, broiled, or microwaved 119
frozen, fillets (*Delta Pride*) 90
frozen, nuggets (*Delta Pride*) 170
frozen, whole (*Delta Pride*) 130

Catsup, see "Ketchup"

Cauliflower:

fresh, raw (*Dole*), ⅙ medium head 25
fresh, boiled, drained, 1″ pieces, ½ cup 14
fresh, green, raw (*Dole*), ⅕ head 35
fresh, green, boiled, drained, 1″ pieces, ½ cup 20
frozen (*Birds Eye*), ½ cup 20
frozen, w/carrots and snow pea pods (*Birds Eye*),
   ½ cup 30
frozen, w/carrots, sugar snap peas, and sweet peas
   (*Green Giant American Mixtures*), ¾ cup 35

Cauliflower, pickled, sweet (*Vlasic*), 1 oz. 35

Cavatelli, frozen (*Celentano*), 3.2 oz. 400

Caviar (see also "Roe"), 1 tbsp.:

black or red 40
lumpfish, black or red (*Romanoff*) 15
salmon, red (*Romanoff*) 35
whitefish, black (*Romanoff*) 25

Cayenne, see "Pepper"

Celeriac, fresh, raw, ½ cup 31

Celery, raw (*Dole*), 2 medium stalks, 3.9 oz. 20

Celery, dried, flakes or seed (*Tone's*), 1 tsp. 9

Celery salt (*Tone's*), 1 tsp. 6

Celtus, raw, trimmed, 1 oz. 6

Cereal, ready-to-eat (see also specific grains):

amaranth flakes (*Arrowhead Mills*), 1 cup 130
bran (*Kellogg's All-Bran*), ½ cup 80
bran, raisin (*Kellogg's*), 1 cup 170
bran flakes (*Kellogg's Complete*), ¾ cup 100
corn (*Nut & Honey Crunch*), 1¼ cups 220
corn (*Post Toasties*), 1 cup 100
cornflakes (*Kellogg's Frosted Flakes*), ¾ cup 120

cornflakes (*Total* Corn Flakes), 1⅓ cups 110
granola (*Kellogg's* Lowfat), ½ cup 210
granola, almond (*Sun Country*), ½ cup 270
granola, raisin (*Kellogg's* Low Fat), ⅔ cup 210
granola, raisin and date (*Sun Country*), 1 cup 260
kamut flakes (*Arrowhead Mills*), 1 cup 120
mixed grain (*Apple Jacks*), 1 cup 110
mixed grain (*Basic 4*), 1 cup 210
mixed grain (*Cinnamon Toast Crunch*), ¾ cup 130
mixed grain (*Fiber One*), ½ cup 60
mixed grain (*Golden Grahams*), ¾ cup 120
mixed grain (*Grape-Nuts*), ½ cup 200
mixed grain (*Grape-Nuts* Flakes), ¾ cup 100
mixed grain (*Kellogg's Mueslix* Crispy), ⅔ cup 200
mixed grain (*Kix*), 1⅓ cups 120
mixed grain (*Multi·Grain Cheerios*), 1 cup 110
mixed grain (*Product 19*), 1 cup 110
mixed grain (*Quaker 100% Natural*), ½ cup 220
mixed grain (*Quaker Life*), ¾ cup 120
mixed grain (*Total* Whole Grain), ¾ cup 110
mixed grain (*Trix*), 1 cup 120
oat (*Alpha-Bits*), 1 cup 130
oat (*Apple Cinnamon Cheerios*), ¾ cup 120
oat (*Cheerios*), 1 cup 110
oat (*Frosted Cheerios/Honey Nut Cheerios*), 1 cup 120
oat (*Honey Bunches of Oats*), ¾ cup 120
oat, almonds (*Honey Bunches of Oats*), ¾ cup 130
oat bran (*Cracklin' Oat Bran*), ¾ cup 230
oat bran (*Quaker*), 1¼ cups 210
oatmeal, toasted, plain or honey nut (*Quaker*), 1 cup . . . 190
rice (*Cocoa Krispies*), ¾ cup 120
rice (*Frosted Krispies*), ¾ cup 110
rice (*Rice Krispies*), 1¼ cups 110
rice (*Rice Krispies Treats*), ¾ cup 120
rice, puffed (*Quaker*), 1 cup 50
rice and corn, almond raisin (*Nutri-Grain*), 1¼ cups . . . 200
spelt flakes (*Arrowhead Mills*), 1 cup 100
wheat (*Clusters*), 1 cup 210
wheat (*Kellogg's Frosted Mini-Wheats*), 1 cup 190
wheat (*Wheaties*), 1 cup 110

Cereal, ready-to-eat *(cont.)*

wheat, puffed (*Quaker*), 1 cup 50

wheat, shredded (*Quaker*), 3 pieces 220

Cereal, cooking, uncooked:

barley, banana nut (*Fantastic* Cup), 1.6 oz. 170

farina, see "wheat," below

mixed grain (*Mothers*), ½ cup 130

mixed grain (*Quaker*), ½ cup 130

mixed grain, maple raisin (*Fantastic* Cup), 1.8 oz. 180

mixed grain, strawberry banana (*Fantastic* Cup),

    1.7 oz. 180

oat bran (*Mothers*), ½ cup 150

oat bran (*Quaker*), ½ cup 150

oat bran, mango (*Fantastic* Cup), 1.8 oz. 180

oatmeal, instant, 1 pkt., except as noted:

    (*Quaker*) 100

    apple cinnamon (*Fantastic* Cup), 1.7 oz. 170

    apples and cinnamon or cinnamon toast (*Quaker*) . . . 130

    bananas and cream (*Quaker*) 140

    blueberries and cream or peaches and cream

      (*Quaker*) 130

    cinnamon spice (*Quaker*) 170

    cranberry orange (*Fantastic* Cup), 1.7 oz. 180

    maple brown sugar or raisin spice (*Quaker*) 160

    raisin, date, and walnut (*Quaker*) 140

oats (*H-O* Quick), ½ cup 150

oats, rolled (*Quaker* Quick/Old Fashioned), ½ cup 150

oats, toasted (*H-O* Old Fashioned), ⅓ cup 160

rice (*Arrowhead Mills Rice & Shine*), ¼ cup 150

rice, all varieties, except sweet almond (*Lundberg* Hot 'n

    Creamy), ⅓ cup 190

rice, almond, sweet (*Lundberg* Hot 'n Creamy), ⅓ cup . . 200

rye, cream of (*Roman Meal*), 1 pkt. 110

wheat (*Mothers*), ½ cup 130

wheat (*Wheatena*), ⅓ cup 150

wheat n' berries (*Fantastic* Cup), 1.7 oz. 170

wheat and oat, peachberry (*Fantastic* Cup), 1.8 oz. 190

wheat, farina (*H-O*), 3 tbsp. 120

Cereal bar, see "Granola and cereal bar"

Chayote:
raw (*Frieda's*), 3.5 oz. 28
boiled, drained, 1″ pieces, ½ cup 19
Cheese (see also "Cheese food," "Cheese product," and
"Cheese Spread"):
American, processed (*Boar's Head* Loaf), 1 oz. 100
American, processed (*Kraft* Deluxe Slice), 1-oz. slice . . . 110
American, processed, sharp (*Borden*), 1 oz. 110
(*Bel Paese*) flavored varieties, 1 oz. 110
blue (*Kraft*), 1 oz. 100
brick (*Kraft*), 1 oz. 110
butterkase, plain or smoked (*Boar's Head*), 1 oz. 100
cheddar (*Cracker Barrel*), 1 oz. 110
cheddar (*Cracker Barrel* ⅓ Less Fat), 1 oz. 80
cheddar, mild or sharp (*Kraft* ⅓ Less Fat), 1 oz. 80
cheddar, nacho, w/peppers (*Kraft*), 1 oz. 110
cheddar, shredded (*Kraft*), ¼ cup 120
cheddar, shredded, mild (*Kraft* ⅓ Less Fat), ¼ cup 90
cheddar, shredded, sharp (*Cracker Barrel* ⅓ Less Fat),
  ¼ cup 80
Cheshire, 1 oz. 110
Colby (*Kraft*), 1 oz. 110
Colby (*Kraft* ⅓ Less Fat), 1 oz. 80
Colby Monterey Jack (*Kraft*), 1 oz. 110
Colby Monterey Jack, shredded (*Kraft*), ¼ cup 120
cottage, 4%, California style (*Friendship*), ½ cup 115
cottage, 4%, w/pineapple (*Friendship*), ½ cup 140
cottage, 2% or 1% (*Weight Watchers*), ½ cup 90
cottage, 1% (*Friendship/Friendship* Low Sodium),
  ½ cup 90
cottage, low-fat, w/pineapple (*Friendship*), ½ cup 120
cottage, nonfat (*Friendship*), ½ cup 80
cottage, nonfat, w/peach (*Friendship*), ½ cup 110
cream cheese (*Boar's Head*), 1 oz. 100
cream cheese (*Weight Watchers* Light), 2 tbsp. 40
cream cheese, reduced fat (*Friendship*), 1 oz. 50
cream cheese, soft (*Friendship*), 2 tbsp. 100
cream cheese, whipped (*Temp-Tee*), 3 tbsp. 110
Edam (*Dorman* Sliced), 1 oz. 90
farmer (*Kraft*), 1 oz. 100

Cheese *(cont.)*

feta (*Alpine Lace* Reduced Fat), 1 oz. 60
fontina (*Classica*), 1 oz. 110
goat, hard type, 1 oz. 128
goat, semisoft type, 1 oz. 103
goat, soft type, 1 oz. 76
Gorgonzola (*Galbani* Dolcelatte), 1 oz. 93
Gouda (*Kraft*), 1 oz. 110
Gruyère, 1 oz. 117
Havarti (*Kraft Casino*), 1 oz. 120
hot pepper (*Alpine Lace*), 1 oz. 80
Italian blend, shredded (*Heluva* Good), ¼ cup 90
Italian style, grated (*Kraft* ⅓ Less Fat), 2 tsp. 25
Jarlsberg (*Sargento*), 1.2-oz. slice 120
(*Laughing Cow* Original Wedge), 1 oz. 70
Limburger (*Kraft Mohawk Valley*), 1 oz. 90
mascarpone (*Classica* Domestic), 1 oz. 120
Monterey Jack (*Kraft*), 1 oz. 110
Monterey Jack (*Kraft* ⅓ Less Fat), 1 oz. 80
Monterey Jack, shredded (*Kraft*), ¼ cup 110
Monterey Jack, jalapeño (*Kraft*), 1 oz. 110
Monterey Jack, peppers (*Kraft* ⅓ Less Fat), 1 oz. 80
mozzarella, whole milk (*Polly-O*), 1 oz. 80
mozzarella, part skim (*Kraft*), 1 oz. 80
mozzarella, shredded, whole milk (*Kraft*), ¼ cup 90
mozzarella, shredded, part skim (*Kraft*), ¼ cup 90
mozzarella, shredded, part skim (*Kraft* ⅓ Less Fat),
    ¼ cup 80
Muenster (*Alpine Lace* Reduced Sodium), 1 oz. 100
Muenster (*Kraft*), 1 oz. 110
Neufchâtel (*Philadelphia Brand*), 1 oz. 70
Parmesan, grated (*Kraft* Italian Blend), 2 tsp. 25
Parmesan, grated or shredded (*Kraft*), 2 tsp. 20
Parmesan-Romano, grated (*Sargento*), 1 tbsp. 25
pimiento, processed (*Kraft* Deluxe), 1 oz. 100
pizza, shredded, all varieties except mozzarella and
    cheddar (*Kraft*), ¼ cup 90
pizza, shredded, mozzarella and cheddar (*Kraft*), ¼ cup   100
Port du Salut, 1 oz. 100
provolone (*Dorman*), 1 oz. 100

provolone, smoke flavor (*Kraft*), 1 oz. 100
ricotta (*Breakstone's*), ¼ cup 110
ricotta, part skim (*Polly-O*), ¼ cup 90
Romano, grated (*Kraft*), 2 tsp. 25
Romano-Parmesan, grated (*Polly-O*), 2 tsp. 25
Roquefort, 1 oz. 105
string (*Polly-O*), 1 oz. 80
string (*Polly-O* Light Mozzarella), 1 oz. 60
Swiss (*Kraft*), 1 oz. 110
Swiss, baby (*Cracker Barrel*), 1 oz. 110
Swiss, processed (*Kraft* Deluxe), 1-oz. slice 90
Swiss, shredded (*Kraft*), ¼ cup 110
taco, shredded, cheddar/Monterey Jack (*Kraft*), ¼ cup . . 100
(*Tal-Fino* Taleggio), 1 oz. 110
"Cheese," substitute and nondairy:
(*Sandwich-Mate*), .7-oz. slice 60
all varieties, (*Weight Watchers* Fat Free), ¾-oz. slice 30
American flavor or Swiss (*Borden*), 1 slice 60
cheddar flavor (*Borden/Bordern* Taco Mate), 1 oz. 100
grated Italian topping (*Weight Watchers*), 1 tbsp. 20
Monterey Jack (*Borden*), 1 oz. 90
mozzarella, shredded (*Borden*), ¼ cup 90
Cheese dip, 2 tbsp.:
and bacon (*Nalley*) 110
blue (*Kraft* Premium) 45
cheddar, mild (*Frito-Lay*) 50
cheddar and mustard (*Heluva* Good Pretzel) 80
chili (*Fritos*) 45
nacho (*Kraft* Premium) 60
salsa (*Old El Paso*) 40
salsa (*Old El Paso Low Fat*) 30
Cheese food (see also "Cheese," "Cheese product," and
   "Cheese spread"):
all varieties (*Kraft* Singles), ¾-oz. slice 70
all varieties, shredded (*Velveeta/Velveeta* Mexican),
   ¼ cup 130
American, grated (*Kraft*), 1 tbsp. 25
cheddar, sharp or extra sharp (*Cracker Barrel*), 2 tbsp. 100
w/garlic or jalapeños (*Kraft*), 1 oz. 90
port wine (*Wispride* Cup), 2 tbsp. 100

Cheese food *(cont.)*
port wine (*Wispride* Light Cup), 2 tbsp. 80
smoke flavor (*Kaukauna* Smokey), 1 oz. 90
smoke flavor (*Kaukauna Lite 50* Smokey), 1 oz. 70
Cheese loaf, American, processed (*Borden*), 1 oz. 110
Cheese product (see also "Cheese food" and "Cheese
  spread"):
(*Cheez Whiz Light*), 2 tbsp. 80
(*Velveeta Light*), 1 oz. 60
all varieties (*Alpine Lace* Nonfat), 1 oz. 45
all varieties (*Kraft Free* Singles), ¾-oz. slice 30
Cheese sauce:
(*Cheez Whiz* Squeezable), 2 tbsp. 100
(*Cheez Whiz Zap-A-Pack* Original/Salsa), 2 tbsp. 90
(*Franco-American*), ¼ cup 40
Cheese sauce mix:
(*Durkee*), ¼ pkg. 25
four (*Knorr*), ⅓ pkg. 70
nacho (*Durkee*), ⅕ pkg. 25
Cheese spread (see also "Cheese," "Cheese food," and
  "Cheese product"):
all varieties (*Cheez Whiz*), 2 tbsp. 90
all varieties (*Easy Cheese*), 2 tbsp. 100
all varieties (*Heluva* Good), 2 tbsp. 90
all varieties (*Velveeta/Velveeta Italiana*/Mexican), 1 oz. . . . 80
w/bacon (*Kraft*), 2 tbsp. 90
blue cheese (*Kraft Roka*), 2 tbsp. 80
w/jalapeños (*Kraft*), 1 oz. 80
olive and pimiento or pineapple (*Kraft*), 2 tbsp. 70
pimiento (*Kraft*), 2 tbsp. 80
sharp (*Old English*), 2 tbsp. 90
Cheese stick (*Goya* Surullitos), 7 pieces 300
Cheeseburger, see "Beef sandwich"
Cherimoya (*Frieda's*), 3.5 oz. 94
Cherries jubilee (*Lucky Leaf/Musselman's*), ¼ cup 80
Cherry, ½ cup, except as noted:
fresh, sour, red, w/pits 26
fresh, sweet, w/pits 52
canned:
  royal Anne (*Comstock*) 110

   royal Anne (*S&W*) 140
   sour, red, pitted, in water (*Comstock*) 50
   sour, red, pitted, in heavy syrup (*Comstock*) 140
   sweet, dark, pitted, in heavy syrup (*Comstock*) 110
   sweet, dark, pitted, in heavy syrup (*Del Monte*) 120
dried, pitted (*Sonoma*), ¼ cup 140
frozen, unsweetened, dark, sweet (*Big Valley*), ¾ cup . . . 90
Cherry, maraschino (*Haddon House*), 1 piece 10
Cherry drink, 8 fl. oz.:
(*After the Fall* Very Cherry) 100
(*Farmer's Market*) 120
Cherry juice, 8 fl. oz., except as noted:
(*Minute Maid* Box), 8.45 oz. 130
black (*Heinke's/R. W. Knudsen*) 180
blend (*Apple & Eve Nothin' But Juice*) 120
nectar (*Santa Cruz*) 110
Cherry pastry, 1 piece:
dumpling, frozen (*Pepperidge Farm*) 280
pocket (*Tastykake*) 370
Cherry syrup, black (*Fox's*), 2 tbsp. 80
Chestnut, European, roasted, peeled, 1 cup 350
Chicken, fresh, 4 oz., except as noted:
broiler-fryer, roasted:
   w/skin, ½ chicken, 10.5 oz. (15.8 oz. w/bone) 715
   w/skin 271
   meat only 215
   meat only, chopped or diced, 1 cup 266
   skin only, 1 oz. 129
   dark meat only 232
   light meat only 196
   breast, w/skin, ½ breast, 3.5 oz. (8.5 oz. w/bone) . . . 193
   drumstick, w/skin, 1.8 oz. (2.9 oz. w/bone) 112
   leg, w/skin (5.7 oz. w/bone) 265
   thigh, w/skin, 2.2 oz. (2.9 oz. w/bone) 153
   wing, w/skin, 1.2 oz. (2.3 oz. w/bone) 99
capon, roasted, w/skin, ½ capon, 1.4 lb. (2 lb.
   w/bone) 1,457
capon, roasted, w/skin 260
Cornish hen, see "Cornish hen"

Chicken *(cont.)*
roaster, roasted, w/skin, ½ chicken, 1 lb. (1.5 lb.
w/bone) 1,071
roaster, roasted, w/skin 253
stewing, stewed:
w/skin, ½ chicken, 9.2 oz. (13.5 oz. w/bone) 744
w/skin 323
meat only 269
meat only, chopped or diced, 1 cup 332
Chicken, canned, chunk, 2 oz.:
(Hormel) 70
breast (*Hormel/Hormel* No Salt) 60
in broth (*Swanson* Mixin') 110
in water (*Swanson* Premium) 70
Chicken, ground, cooked (*Perdue*), 3 oz. 170
Chicken, refrigerated or frozen:
whole, cooked:
dark meat (*Perdue*), 3 oz. 210
dark meat (*Perdue Oven Stuffer*), 3 oz. 200
white meat (*Perdue/Perdue Oven Stuffer*), 3 oz. 160
barbecued (*Empire* Kosher), 5 oz. edible 280
breast:
raw, halves (*Tyson*), 4 oz. 190
raw, halves, skinless (*Tyson*), 4 oz. 140
raw, quarters (*Tyson*), 4 oz. 210
raw, boneless (*Tyson/Tyson* Tenderloins), 4 oz. 110
raw, boneless, thin sliced (*Perdue*), 3 oz. 80
raw, barbecue (*Perdue*), 4 oz. 130
raw, lemon pepper or Italian (*Perdue*), 4 oz. 110
raw, Oriental (*Perdue*), 4 oz. 120
cooked, whole (*Perdue*), 3 oz. 160
cooked, whole (*Perdue Oven Stuffer*), 3 oz. 150
cooked, boneless (*Perdue/Perdue Oven Stuffer*),
3 oz. 120
cooked, quartered (*Perdue*), 3 oz. 180
cooked, roundelet (*Tyson*), 2.6-oz. piece 170
cooked, tenderloins (*Perdue*), 3 oz. 100
cooked, thin sliced (*Perdue*), 2 oz. 80
cooked, white meat roll (*Tyson*), 2 slices, 1.3 oz. 60
cooked, boneless, barbecue (*Perdue*), 3 oz. 110

cooked, boneless, lemon pepper (*Perdue*), 3 oz. 90
cooked, boneless, Italian or Oriental (*Perdue*),
  3 oz. 100
fried, battered and breaded (*Empire* Kosher), 3 oz.
  edible 170
roasted (*Perdue*), 6.7-oz. half 370
roasted (*Tyson*), ½ breast 250
roasted, boneless (*Perdue*), 3.6-oz. half 140
roasted, boneless (*Perdue Fit 'n Easy*), 3.6-oz. half . . 150
roasted, skinless (*Perdue*), 5.9-oz. half 250
chunks, cooked (*Tyson Chick'n Chunks*), 6 pieces,
  3 oz. 280
cutlet, battered, breaded (*Empire* Kosher),
  3.3-oz. piece 200
diced (*Tyson*), 3 oz. 130
drum and thigh, fried (*Empire* Kosher), 3 oz. edible 240
drumstick, roasted (*Perdue*), 2.2-oz. piece 110
drumstick, roasted (*Perdue Oven Stuffer*),
  3.6-oz. piece 190
drumstick, roasted (*Tyson*), 3 pieces 330
drumstick, roasted, skinless (*Perdue* Pick), 2 pieces,
  3.5 oz. 150
drumsticks, thighs, and wings, raw (*Tyson* Multipak),
  4 oz. 230
frying parts (*Tyson*), 4 oz. 250
gizzards, raw (*Tyson*), 4 oz. 90
half, roasted, w/out skin (*Tyson*), 3 oz. 140
leg, whole, roasted (*Perdue*), 5.5 oz. 370
leg, whole, roasted (*Perdue* Jumbo Family/Value), 5.5 oz. 360
leg, quarters, raw (*Tyson*), 4 oz. 290
leg, quarters, cooked (*Perdue*), 3 oz. 210
nuggets (*Empire* Kosher), 5 pieces, 3 oz. 180
patties, breaded, w/cheddar (*Tyson Chick'n with*
  Cheddar), 1 piece 220
sticks (*Empire* Kosher Stix), 4 pieces, 3.1 oz. 180
thigh, raw (*Tyson*), 4 oz. 250
thigh, raw, boneless, skinless (*Tyson/Tyson* Jumbo),
  4 oz. 160
thigh, roasted (*Perdue*), 3.2-oz. piece 240
thigh, roasted (*Tyson*), 3.6-oz. piece 270

Chicken, refrigerated or frozen *(cont.)*

thigh, roasted, boneless (*Perdue*), 2 pieces, 3.6 oz. 200
thigh, roasted, boneless (*Perdue Fit 'n Easy*), 2 pieces . . 190
thigh, roasted, boneless (*Perdue Oven Stuffer*),
   3.3 oz. 170
thigh, roasted, skinless (*Perdue*), 2.7 oz. 160
wing, raw, whole (*Tyson*), 4 oz. 250
wing, roasted (*Perdue*), 2 pieces 210
wing, roasted (*Perdue* Wingettes), 3 pieces 200
wing, roasted (*Perdue Oven Stuffer* Drummettes),
   2 pieces 170
wing, roasted (*Perdue Oven Stuffer* Wingettes), 3 pieces 220
"Chicken," vegetarian:
canned, diced (*Worthington* Chik), ¼ cup 60
canned, fried (*Worthington FriChik*), 2 pieces 120
canned, fried, w/gravy (*Loma Linda Chik'n*), 2 pieces . . . 210
frozen (*Worthington Chik-Stiks*), 1 piece 110
frozen, fried (*Loma Linda Chik'n*), 1 piece 180
frozen, nuggets (*Loma Linda*), 5 pieces 240
frozen, patties (*Worthington Crispy Chik*), 1 patty 170
frozen, roll or sliced (*Worthington*), 2 slices 80
Chicken dinner, frozen:
barbecue, mesquite (*The Budget Gourmet*), 11 oz. 270
barbecue, mesquite (*Healthy Choice*), 10.5 oz. 270
barbecue, w/potato and vegetables (*Tyson* BBQ),
   1 pkg. 560
breaded, country (*Healthy Choice*), 10¼ oz. 360
breast, 11 oz.:
   herbed, w/fettuccine (*The Budget Gourmet*) 260
   honey mustard (*The Budget Gourmet*) 310
   roasted, w/herb gravy (*The Budget Gourmet*) 250
broccoli Alfredo (*Healthy Choice*), 11.5 oz. 300
cacciatore (*Healthy Choice*), 12.5 oz. 250
Cantonese (*Healthy Choice*), 10¾ oz. 260
Dijon (*Healthy Choice*), 11 oz. 270
fingers, and BBQ sauce (*Freezer Queen* Meal), 9 oz. . . . 310
Francesca (*Healthy Choice*), 12.5 oz. 330
fried, Southern (*Banquet* Extra Helping), 17.5 oz. 750
ginger, Hunan (*Healthy Choice*), 12.6 oz. 350
grilled, Southwestern (*Healthy Choice*), 10.2 oz. 200

herb, country (*Healthy Choice*), 12.15 oz. 310
nuggets (*Freezer Queen* Meal), 6 oz. 320
parmigiana (*The Budget Gourmet*), 11 oz. 280
patty (*Freezer Queen* Meal), 7.5 oz. 290
picante (*Healthy Choice*), 10.75 oz. 260
roasted (*Healthy Choice*), 11 oz. 220
sesame, Shanghai (*Healthy Choice*), 12 oz. 310
sweet and sour (*Healthy Choice*), 11 oz. 330
teriyaki (*The Budget Gourmet*), 11 oz. 300
teriyaki (*Healthy Choice*), 11 oz. 230
Chicken entree, canned:
à la king (*Top Shelf*), 10 oz. 380
breast, glazed (*Top Shelf*), 10 oz. 200
cacciatore (*Top Shelf*), 10 oz. 210
chow mein (*La Choy* Bi-Pack), 1 cup 110
chow mein (*La Choy* Entree), 1 cup 80
and dumplings (*Dinty Moore* Cup), 7½ oz. 190
fiesta (*Top Shelf*), 10 oz. 420
and noodles (*Dinty Moore American Classics*), 10 oz. . . 260
noodles and, see "Noodle entree"
Oriental, w/noodles (*La Choy*), 1 cup 150
and pasta (*Chef Boyardee* Bowl), 7½ oz. 150
w/potatoes (*Dinty Moore American Classics*), 10 oz. . . . 220
spicy (*La Choy* Szechwan Bi-Pack), 1 cup 100
stew (*Dinty Moore*), 1 cup 220
sweet and sour (*La Choy* Bi-Pack), 1 cup 160
teriyaki (*La Choy* Bi-Pack), 1 cup 110
Chicken entree, frozen:
à la king (*Freezer Queen* Cook-in-Pouch), 4-oz. pkg. . . . 70
à la king (*Stouffer's*), 9.5 oz. 350
au gratin (*The Budget Gourmet* Light), 9.1 oz. 250
baked, w/potato and stuffing (*Lean Cuisine*), 8.5 oz. . . . 250
barbecue (*Tyson*), 8.9 oz. 270
w/basil cream sauce (*Lean Cuisine Cafe Classics*), 8.5 oz. 260
and biscuits (*Freezer Queen* Family), 1 cup, 7.9 oz. 210
blackened, w/rice and corn (*Tyson*), 8.9 oz. 260
breast, in wine sauce (*Lean Cuisine* Cafe Classics),
    8⅛ oz. 220
breast, stuffed, 6-oz. piece:
    asparagus and cheese (*Barber Foods*) 350

Chicken entree, frozen, breast, stuffed *(cont.)*
    broccoli and cheese (*Barber Foods*) 330
    Cordon Bleu (*Barber Foods*) 360
    Kiev (*Barber Foods*) 420
    skinless (*Barber Foods*) 300
breast tenders (*Tyson*), 5 pieces, 3 oz. 220
breast tenders, regular or Southern (*Banquet*), 3 pieces,
    3 oz. 260
and broccoli (*Healthy Choice Hearty Handfuls*), 6.1 oz. . . 320
w/broccoli and cheese (*Tyson*), 8.9 oz. 270
cacciatore (*Tyson*), 14.9 oz. 560
calypso (*Lean Cuisine* Cafe Classics), 8.5 oz. 280
carbonara (*Lean Cuisine* Cafe Classics), 9 oz. 280
chow mein (*Lean Cuisine*), 9 oz. 240
chow mein (*Smart Ones*), 9 oz. 200
chunks, breaded (*Country Skillet*), 5 pieces, 3.3 oz. . . . 270
chunks, breaded, Southern (*Country Skillet*), 5 pieces,
    3.3 oz. 250
Cordon Bleu (*Weight Watchers*), 9 oz. 230
creamed (*Stouffer's*), 6.5 oz. 260
creamy, and broccoli (*Stouffer's*), 8⅞ oz. 320
croquette (*Tyson*), 3.5 oz. 290
croquette, gravy and (*Freezer Queen* Family),
    ⅙ of 28-oz. pkg. 140
enchilada, see "Enchilada entree"
escalloped, and noodles (*Stouffer's*), 10 oz. 450
fettuccine (*The Budget Gourmet*), 10 oz. 380
fettuccine (*Lean Cuisine*), 9¼ oz. 300
fettuccine (*Weight Watchers*), 10 oz. 290
fettuccine Alfredo (*Healthy Choice*), 8.5 oz. 260
fiesta (*Lean Cuisine*), 8.5 oz. 250
fiesta (*Smart Ones*), 8.5 oz. 220
French recipe (*The Budget Gourmet* Light), 9 oz. 180
fricassee w/rice (*Goya*), 1 pkg. 810
fried, w/mashed potatoes, gravy (*Tyson*), 10.9 oz. 360
fried, w/whipped potato (*Stouffer's* Homestyle),
    7.5 oz. 310
fried pieces:
    breast (*Banquet*), 5.5-oz. piece 410
    drums and thighs or hot 'n spicy (*Banquet*), 3 oz. . . . 260

original, country, or Southern (*Banquet*), 3 oz. 270
  skinless, original, or honey BBQ (*Banquet*), 3 oz. . . . 210
  wing, hot and spicy (*Banquet*), 4 oz., 4 pieces 230
garlic (*Healthy Choice Hearty Handfuls*), 6.1 oz. 330
garlic, Milano (*Healthy Choice*), 9.5 oz. 240
glazed (*Stouffer's* 63 oz.), 4.2 oz. 100
glazed, country (*Healthy Choice*), 8.5 oz. 210
glazed, w/rice, broccoli, and carrots (*Tyson*), 9.1 oz. . . . 240
glazed, w/vegetable rice (*Lean Cuisine*), 8.5 oz. 240
grilled (*Healthy Choice* Sonoma), 9 oz. 240
grilled, and angel-hair pasta (*Stouffer's*), 10⁷/₈ oz. 380
grilled, w/corn and beans (*Tyson*), 8.9 oz. 240
grilled, Italian, w/linguini (*Tyson*), 8.9 oz. 190
grilled, w/mashed potatoes (*Healthy Choice*), 8 oz. 170
grilled, salsa (*Lean Cuisine* Cafe Classics), 8⁷/₈ oz. 270
honey mustard (*Tyson*), 11.35 oz. 340
imperial, w/rice (*Freezer Queen* Homestyle), 9 oz. 250
mandarin (*The Budget Gourmet* Light), 10 oz. 270
mandarin (*Lean Cuisine Lunch Classics*), 9 oz. 260
marinara rotini (*Lean Cuisine Lunch Classics*), 9.5 oz. . . 260
Marsala (*The Budget Gourmet*), 9 oz. 270
Marsala, w/potato and carrots (*Tyson*), 8.9 oz. 180
Marsala, and vegetables (*Healthy Choice*), 11.5 oz. 230
Mediterranean (*Lean Cuisine* Cafe Classics), 10.5 oz. . . . 230
mesquite (*Tyson*), 8.9 oz. 320
w/mushroom sauce (*Tyson*), 8.9 oz. 220
and noodles (*The Budget Gourmet*), 9 oz. 380
nuggets (*Country Skillet*), 10 pieces, 3.3 oz. 280
nuggets (*Freezer Queen* Family), 6 pieces, 3 oz. 240
nuggets, mozzarella (*Banquet*), 6 pieces, 2.9 oz. 250
orange glazed (*The Budget Gourmet* Light), 9 oz. 300
Oriental (*The Budget Gourmet* Light), 9 oz. 300
Oriental (*Lean Cuisine*), 9 oz. 250
parmigiana (*Banquet* Family), 4.7-oz. piece 240
parmigiana (*Stouffer's* Homestyle), 12 oz. 460
parmigiana (*Tyson*), 13.8 oz. 430
parmigiana, Italian style (*Banquet*), 4.6-oz. piece 250
patties, breaded (*Country Skillet*), 2¹/₂-oz. patty 190
patties, breaded, Southern (*Country Skillet*), 3.3-oz. patty 190
piccata (*Lean Cuisine* Cafe Classics), 9 oz. 270

Chicken entree, frozen *(cont.)*

piccata, lemon herb (*Smart Ones*), 8.5 oz.	200
piccata, w/potato and broccoli (*Tyson*), 8.9 oz.	190

pie/potpie:

(*Banquet*), 7-oz. pie	350
(*Lean Cuisine*), 9.5 oz.	310
(*Marie Callender's*), 10-oz. pie	680
(*Stouffer's*), 10-oz. pie	560
(*Tyson/Tyson* All Meat), 8.9 oz.	470
au gratin (*Marie Callender's*), 10-oz. pie	720
and broccoli (*Marie Callender's*), 10-oz. pie	780
primavera, pasta (*Tyson*), 11.35 oz.	320
w/rice (*Goya* Arroz con Pollo), 1 pkg.	750
roasted, herb (*Lean Cuisine* Cafe Classics), 8 oz.	210
roasted, herb (*Tyson*), 11.35 oz.	290
roasted, w/pasta and vegetables (*Tyson*), 8.9 oz.	210
sandwich, see "Chicken sandwich"	
sliced, gravy and (*Freezer Queen* Cook-in-Pouch), 4 oz.	60
sweet and sour (*The Budget Gourmet*), 10 oz.	330
sweet and sour, w/rice (*Freezer Queen*), 9 oz.	240
and vegetables (*Lean Cuisine*), 10.5 oz.	250
and vegetables, w/linguine (*Freezer Queen* Deluxe Family), 1 cup, 8.6 oz.	250
and vegetables, w/noodles (*Freezer Queen*), 9 oz.	210
wings (*Tyson Wings of Fire*), 4 pieces, 3.4 oz.	220
wings, barbecue (*Tyson*), 4 pieces, 3.4 oz.	210

Chicken entree mix:

Alfredo (*Dinner Sensations*), 1 cup*	310
Alfredo, low-fat recipe (*Dinner Sensations*), 1 cup*	300
stir-fry (*Skillet Chicken Helper*), 1 cup*	270
sweet and sour (*Dinner Sensations*), 1 cup*	330

Chicken frankfurter (*Empire* Kosher), 2-oz. link 100

Chicken giblets, simmered, chopped, 1 cup 228

Chicken gravy, ¼ cup:

canned (*Heinz* Home Style Classic)	20
canned (*Heinz* Home Style Fat Free)	15
canned, cream of (*Pepperidge Farm*)	30
canned, rotisserie or golden w/chicken (*Pepperidge Farm*)	25
mix* (*McCormick*)	20

mix* (*Pillsbury* with Water) 10
mix* (*Weight Watchers*) 10
Chicken lunch meat, breast:
all varieties (*Tyson*), 2 slices, 1.5 oz. 35
baked, grilled, or honey glazed (*Louis Rich Carving
    Board*), 2 slices, 1.6 oz. 45
honey glazed (*Oscar Mayer Deli-Thin*), 4 slices, 1.8 oz. . 60
oven roasted (*Louis Rich* Deluxe), 1-oz. slice 30
oven roasted (*Louis Rich Deli-Thin*), 4 slices, 1.8 oz. . . . 50
oven roasted (*Oscar Mayer* Fat Free), 4 slices, 1.8 oz. . . . 45
white, oven roasted (*Louis Rich*), 1-oz. slice 40
Chicken pie, see "Chicken entree, frozen"
Chicken sandwich, frozen, 1 piece:
broccoli supreme (*Lean Pockets*), 4.5-oz. piece 240
broccoli and cheddar (*Croissant Pockets*), 4.5-oz.
    piece 300
and cheddar w/broccoli (*Hot Pockets*), 4.5-oz. piece . . . 300
fajita (*Lean Pockets*), 4.5-oz. piece 260
fajita (*Totino's* Big & Hearty), 4.8-oz. piece 270
grilled (*Tyson* Microwave), 3.45 oz. 210
Parmesan (*Lean Pockets*), 4.5-oz. piece 260
Chicken sauce (see also specific listings):
barbecue flavor (*Hunt's Chicken Sensations*), 1 tbsp. . . . 35
cacciatore (*Ragu Chicken Tonight*), 1/2 cup 80
country French (*Ragu Chicken Tonight*), 1/2 cup 130
creamy, w/mushrooms (*Ragu Chicken Tonight*), 1/2 cup . . 110
creamy, primavera (*Ragu Chicken Tonight*), 1/2 cup 90
Dijon or teriyaki (*Lawry's Chicken Saute*), 2 tbsp. 40
garlic Italian (*Lawry's Chicken Saute*), 2 tbsp. 30
herbed, w/wine (*Ragu Chicken Tonight*), 1/2 cup 80
Italian garlic, lemon herb, or Southwestern (*Hunt's
    Chicken Sensations*), 1 tbsp. 30
lemon herb (*Lawry's Chicken Saute*), 2 tbsp. 25
sweet and sour (*Ragu Chicken Tonight*), 1/2 cup 120
wing (*Stubb's Legendary* Original/Inferno), 1 tbsp. 10
wing, Buffalo (*World Harbors* Hot Zings), 2 tbsp. 30
Chicken sausage, all varieties (*Gerhard's*), 2.5 oz. 110
Chicken seasoning/coating mix:
(*Durkee/French's* Roasting Bag), 1/6 pkg. 20
(*McCormick's Bag 'n Season*), 1 tbsp. 20

Chicken seasoning/coating mix *(cont.)*
barbecue (*Durkee* Roasting Bag), ⅙ pkg. 30
cacciatore or Mexican salsa (*Durkee Easy*), ¹/₁₀ pkg. 10
country (*Durkee* Roasting Bag), ⅙ pkg. 35
hot, spicy (*McCormick Bag 'n Season*), 1 tbsp. 30
mushroom (*Durkee Easy*), ⅛ pkg. 15
sweet and sour (*Durkee Easy*), ⅑ pkg. 20
Chicken spread:
chunky (*Underwood*), ¼ cup 120
chunky, w/crackers (*Red Devil* Snackers), 1 pkg. 280
Chickpeas:
dry (*Arrowhead Mills*), ¼ cup 170
dry, boiled, ½ cup 134
canned (*Green Giant/Joan of Arc*), ½ cup 110
canned (*Progresso*), ½ cup 120
canned (*Progresso* Garbanzo), ½ cup 100
canned (*Seneca* Garbanzo), ½ cup 110
Chicory, witloof, ½ cup 8
Chicory greens, chopped, ½ cup 21
Chicory root, 1″ pieces, ½ cup 33
Chili, canned, 1 cup, except as noted:
w/beans (*Broadcast*) 120
w/beans (*Chi-Chi's* San Antonio) 340
w/beans (*Hormel*) 340
w/beans, cheddar (*Nalley*) 320
w/out beans (*Hormel/Hormel* Hot) 410
w/out beans, onion (*Nalley* Walla Walla) 300
w/franks, see "Beans and franks"
w/macaroni (*Hormel* Chili Mac), 7.5-oz. can 200
turkey, w/beans (*Hormel*) 220
turkey, w/out beans (*Hormel*) 190
Chili, frozen:
three bean (*Lean Cuisine* Entree), 10-oz. pkg. 260
vegetarian (*Tabatchnik* Side Dish), 7.5-oz. pkg. 210
Chili, mix:
all varieties (*Health Valley* Chili in a Cup), ⅓ cup 120
3 bean or vegetarian (*Spice Islands* Quick Meal),
   1 pkg. 180
Chili base, canned:
(*Stubb's Legendary* Chili Fixin's), ½ cup 50

all varieties (*S&W* Chili Makin's), ½ cup 80
Chili beans (see also "Mexican beans"), canned:
(*Stokely*), ½ cup 120
(*Van Camp's* Mexican), ½ cup 110
spicy (*Green Giant/Joan of Arc*), ½ cup 110
Chili dip, green (*La Victoria*), 2 tbsp. 10
Chili dip mix, caliente (*Knorr*), ½ tsp. 5
Chili pepper, see "Pepper, chili"
Chili powder (*Gebhardt*), ¼ tsp. 1
Chili sauce (see also "Pepper sauce"):
(*Del Monte*), 1 tbsp. 20
(*Las Palmas*), ¼ cup 15
hot dog (*Gebhardt*), ¼ cup 60
Chili seasoning mix:
(*Adolph's Meal Makers*), 1 tbsp. 40
(*Gebhardt Chili Quik*), 2 tbsp. 30
(*Old El Paso*), 1 tbsp. 25
Chimichanga, frozen:
beef (*Old El Paso*), 4.3-oz. piece 360
chicken (*Old El Paso*), 4.3-oz. piece 340
Chimichanga dinner, frozen:
beef (*Chi-Chi's*), 15-oz. pkg. 630
chicken (*Chi-Chi's*), 15-oz. pkg. 600
Chimichanga entree, frozen (*Banquet*), 9.5-oz. pkg. . . . 470
Chitterlings, pork, simmered, 4 oz. 344
Chives, fresh, chopped, or freeze-dried, 1 tbsp. 1
Chocolate, see "Candy"
Chocolate, baking:
(*Choco Bake*), ½ oz. 80
bar (*Hershey's*), ½ of 1-oz. bar 90
bar, bittersweet or semisweet (*Hershey's*), ½ oz. 80
bar, semisweet (*Nestlé*), ½ oz. 70
bar, sweet (*Baker's German*), ½ oz. 60
bar, unsweetened or white (*Nestlé*), ½ oz. 80
bits, peanut butter (*Reese's*), 1 tbsp. 70
bits, toffee (*Skor*), 1 tbsp. 70
chips, milk, mint, or semisweet (*Nestlé*), ½ oz. 70
chips, white (*Ghirardelli*), 1 tbsp. 80
chunks (*Hershey's* Semisweet), 6 chunks 80
kisses (*Hershey's* Mini), 11 pieces 80

Chocolate, baking *(cont.)*
semisweet, plain or mint (*Nestlé*), ½ oz. 70
Chocolate-flavor drink mix
(*Nestlé Quik*), 2 tbsp. 90
(*Nestlé Quik* No Sugar), 2 tbsp. 40
shake (*Weight Watchers*), 1 pkt. 80
Chocolate milk, 8 fl. oz.:
(*Crowley's*) 220
low-fat (*Hershey's*) 190
low-fat (*Parmalat*) 180
fat free (*Hershey's*) 130
Chocolate syrup (*Hershey's*), 2 tbsp. 100
Chocolate topping, 2 tbsp.:
dark (*Smucker's Dove*) 130
(*Kraft*) 110
fudge, dark chocolate or hot (*Mrs. Richardson's*) 140
fudge, hot (*Kraft*) 140
fudge, hot (*Mrs. Richardson's* Fat Free) 110
milk (*Smucker's Dove*) 140
Chorizo (*Goya*), 1.6-oz. stick 160
Chow mein, see specific entree listings
Chowchow (*Stubb's Legendary*), ½ cup 70
Churro, cinnamon (*Tio Pepe's*), 1 oz. 110
Chutney, 1 tbsp.:
mango (*Patak's* Major Grey's) 50
tomato, dried (*Sonoma*) 35
Cilantro, see "Coriander"
Cinnamon, ground (*McCormick*), ¼ tsp. 2
Cisco, meat only, raw, 4 oz. 112
Citron, candied, diced (*Paradise/White Swan*), 2 tbsp. . . . 80
Citrus drink, 8 fl. oz.:
punch (*Goya*) 130
punch (*Tree Top* Juice Rivers Box) 130
frozen*, all varieties (*Five Alive*) 110
Citrus salad, in jars, in light syrup (*Sunfresh*), ½ cup . . . 70
Clam:
fresh, meat only, raw, 9 large or 20 small, 6.3 oz. 133
fresh, meat only, boiled, poached, or steamed, 4 oz. . . . 168
canned, baby, whole (*S&W*), 2 oz. 50
canned, chopped (*S&W*), 2 oz. 20

canned, minced (*Progresso*), 2 oz. 60
canned, smoked (*S&W*), 2 oz. 130
fried, frozen (*Gorton's* Crunchy), 3 oz. 260
fried, frozen (*Mrs. Paul's*), 28 pieces, 3 oz. 280
Clam dip, 2 tbsp.:
(*Kraft*) 60
(*Kraft* Premium) 45
Clam sauce, canned, ½ cup:
creamy (*Progresso*) 110
red (*Progresso*) 80
white (*Progresso*) 130
Cocktail sauce, see "Seafood sauce"
Cocoa, baking, unsweetened (*Nestlé* Baking), 1 tbsp. 15
Cocoa mix, hot, 1 pkt.:
(*Swiss Miss*) 140
(*Swiss Miss* Diet) 20
(*Swiss Miss* Fat Free) 50
(*Swiss Miss* Lite) 70
(*Weight Watchers*) 70
Coconut:
fresh, shelled, shredded (*Dole*), 1 cup not packed 283
packaged, flaked (*Mounds*), 2 tbsp. 70
packaged, and almond bits (*Almond Joy*), 2 tbsp. 60
Coconut cream, canned (*Coco Goya*), 1 tbsp. 140
Coconut milk, canned (*Goya*), 1 tbsp. 50
Cod, meat only, 4 oz.:
Atlantic or Pacific, raw 93
Atlantic or Pacific, baked, broiled, or microwaved 119
frozen, Pacific, loins (*Peter Pan*) 90
Cod entree, breaded, frozen (*Van de Kamp's* Light),
    3.98-oz. piece 220
Coffee, brewed, 6 fl. oz. 4
Coffee creamer, see "Creamer, nondairy"
Coffee substitute:
(*Natural Touch Kaffree Roma*), 1 tsp. 10
(*Natural Touch Roma Cappuccino*), 3 tbsp. 50
Coleslaw, salad mix (*Dole*), 3 oz. 25
Collard greens, ½ cup:
fresh, raw, chopped 6
canned (*Stubb's Harvest*) 30

Collard greens *(cont.)*
canned, seasoned (*Sylvia's Restaurant*) 45
Cookie:
almond (*Sunshine* Crescents), 4 pieces, 1.1 oz. 150
almond toast (*Stella D'Oro* Mandel), 2 pieces, 1 oz. 110
animal (*Barnum's Animals*), 12 pieces, 1.1 oz. 140
anisette (*Stella D'Oro* Toast), 3 pieces, 1.2 oz. 130
apple (*Newtons* Fat Free), 2 pieces, 1 oz. 100
apple (*Sunshine* Golden Fruit), .7-oz. piece 80
apple pastry (*Stella D'Oro* Low Sodium), .7-oz. piece 80
apple and raisin bar (*Smart Snackers*), .75 oz. 70
apricot filled (*Archway*), 1-oz. piece 110
apricot-raspberry (*Pepperidge Farm*), 3 pieces, 1.1 oz. . . . 140
arrowroot (*National*), 2-oz. piece 20
banana bran (*Archway* Low Fat), 1.2-oz. piece 120
biscotti, almond (*Pepperidge Farm Caruso*),
    .7-oz. piece 90
blueberry (*Archway*), 1-oz. piece 110
brown edge wafer (*Nabisco*), 5 pieces, 1 oz. 140
butter (*Pepperidge Farm Chessman*), 3 pieces, .9 oz. . . . 120
butter, sandwich, w/fudge (*E. L. Fudge*), 3 pieces, 1.2 oz. 170
caramel, pecan (*Pepperidge Farm*), .9-oz. piece 130
carrot cake (*Archway*), 1-oz. piece 120
cherry cobbler (*Pepperidge Farm*), .6-oz. piece 70
cherry, filled (*Archway*), 1-oz. piece 110
chocolate:
    (*Stella D'Oro* Castelets), 2 pieces, 1 oz. 130
    (*Stella D'Oro* Margherite), 2 pieces, 1.1 oz. 150
    brownie (*Entenmann's* Fat Free), 2 pieces 80
    brownie nut (*Pepperidge Farm*), 3 pieces, 1.1 oz. . . . 160
    dark (*Pepperidge Farm* Espirits Noir), .6-oz. piece 90
    fudge (*SnackWell's*), 1 oz. 90
    fudge mint (*Grasshopper*), 4 pieces, 1.1 oz. 150
    laced (*Pepperidge Farm Pirouette*), 5 pieces,
        1.2 oz. 180
    w/nuts (*Pepperidge Farm Geneva*), 3 pieces,
        1.1 oz. 160
    orange (*Pepperidge Farm* Chocolat à l'Orange),
        2 pieces, 1.1 oz. 150
    wafer, light (*Keebler*), 8 pieces, 1.1 oz. 130

chocolate chip/chunk:
    (*Entenmann's*), 3 pieces, 1.1 oz. 140
    (*Pepperidge Farm* Old Fashioned), 3 pieces, 1 oz. . . . 140
    (*Pepperidge Farm Chesapeake*), .9-oz. piece 140
    (*Pepperidge Farm Goldfish*), 1.1 oz. 150
    (*Pepperidge Farm Nantucket*), .9-oz. piece 130
    (*Smart Snackers*), 2 pieces, 1.06 oz. 140
    (*SnackWell's* Reduced Fat), 13 pieces, 1 oz. 130
    chocolate, walnut, soft (*Pepperidge Farm*),
      .9-oz. piece 130
    drop (*Archway*), 1-oz. piece 140
    macadamia (*Pepperidge Farm Sausalito*), .9-oz. piece 140
    macadamia, white chunk (*Pepperidge Farm Tahoe*),
      .9-oz. piece 130
    and toffee (*Archway*), 1-oz. piece 140
    toffee (*Pepperidge Farm Charleston*), .9-oz. piece . . . 130
    walnut (*Pepperidge Farm Beacon Hill*), .9-oz. piece . . 130
chocolate sandwich:
    (*E. L. Fudge*), 2 pieces, .9 oz. 120
    (*Elfin Delights* Light), 2 pieces, .9 oz. 110
    (*Hydrox*), 3 pieces, 1.1 oz. 150
    (*Hydrox* Fat Free), 3 pieces, 1.1 oz. 130
    (*Oreo*), 3 pieces, 1.2 oz. 160
    (*Oreo* Reduced Fat), 3 pieces, 1.1 oz. 140
    (*Pepperidge Farm Bordeaux*), 4 pieces, 1 oz. 130
    (*Pepperidge Farm Brussels*), 3 pieces, 1.1 oz. 150
    (*Pepperidge Farm Lido*), .6-oz. piece 90
    (*Pepperidge Farm Milano*), 3 pieces, 1.2 oz. 180
    (*Smart Snackers*), 2 pieces, 1.06 oz. 140
    (*SnackWell's* Reduced Fat), 2 pieces, .9 oz. 100
    double (*Pepperidge Farm Milano*), 2 pieces, 1 oz. . . . 150
    hazelnut (*Pepperidge Farm Milano*), 2 pieces,
      .9 oz. 130
    milk (*Pepperidge Farm Bordeaux*), 3 pieces,
      1.1 oz. 160
    milk (*Pepperidge Farm Milano*), 3 pieces, 1.3 oz. . . . 180
    mint (*Pepperidge Farm Brussels*), 3 pieces, 1.3 oz. . . 190
    mint (*Pepperidge Farm Milano*), 2 pieces, .9 oz. 140
    orange (*Pepperidge Farm Milano*), 2 pieces, .9 oz. . . . 140
cinnamon snaps (*Archway*), 5 pieces, 1.1 oz. 150

Cookie *(cont.)*

coconut (*Dare Breaktime*), .3-oz. piece 35
cranberry bar (*Archway* Fat Free), .75-oz. bar 70
devil's food cake (*SnackWell's* Fat Free), .6-oz. piece 50
fig (*Fig Newtons*), 2 pieces, 1.1 oz. 110
fig (*Smart Snackers*), .7 oz. 70
fortune (*La Choy*), 4 pieces, 1.1 oz. 110
fudge, double, cake (*SnackWell's* Fat Free),
   .6-oz. piece 50
fudge, fudge filled (*Keebler* Truffles), 3 pieces, 1.2 oz. . . 180
ginger (*Pepperidge Farm* Gingerman), 4 pieces, 1 oz. . . . 120
ginger snaps (*Nabisco*), 4 pieces, 1 oz. 120
golden bar (*Stella D'Oro*), 1-oz. piece 110
graham (*Keebler*), 8 pieces, 1 oz. 130
graham, cinnamon (*SnackWell's* Fat Free Snacks),
   20 pieces, 1.1 oz. 110
graham, cinnamon (*Sunshine*), 2 pieces, 1.1 oz. 140
graham, fudge coated (*Keebler* Deluxe), 3 pieces 140
graham, honey (*Sunshine*), 2 pieces, 1 oz. 120
hazelnut (*Pepperidge Farm*), 3 pieces, 1.1 oz. 160
kichel (*Stella D'Oro* Low Sodium), 21 pieces, 1 oz. 150
lemon creme (*Dare*), .7-oz. piece 95
lemon nut crunch (*Pepperidge Farm*), 3 pieces,
   1.1 oz. 170
marshmallow, chocolate (*Mallomars*), 2 pieces, .9 oz. . . 120
mint sandwich (*Mystic Mint*), .6-oz. piece 90
molasses (*Archway*), 1-oz. piece 110
molasses, crisps (*Pepperidge Farm*), 5 pieces, 1.1 oz. . . 150
oatmeal (*Keebler* Classic Collection), 2 pieces, 1 oz. . . . 150
oatmeal (*Sunshine* Country), 3 pieces, 1.2 oz. 170
oatmeal, butterscotch (*Pepperidge Farm*), 3 pieces,
   1.2 oz. 170
oatmeal, chocolate chip (*Sunshine*), 3 pieces, 1.3 oz. . . . 170
oatmeal, Irish (*Pepperidge Farm*), 3 pieces, 1 oz. 130
oatmeal raisin (*Pepperidge Farm* Old Fashioned),
   3 pieces, 1.2 oz. 160
oatmeal raisin (*Pepperidge Farm* Soft), .9 oz. piece 110
oatmeal raisin (*Pepperidge Farm* Santa Fe), .9-oz. piece   120
oatmeal raisin (*Smart Snackers*), 2 pieces, 1.06 oz. 120
oatmeal raisin (*SnackWell's* Reduced Fat), 2 pieces, 1 oz. 110

peach tart (*Pepperidge Farm*), 2 pieces, 1.1 oz. 120
peanut butter fudge (*P. B. Fudgebutters*), 2 pieces, .8 oz. 130
peanut butter graham (*Mr. Peanut P. B. Crisps*),
  1 oz. 140
peanut butter patties (*Nutter Butter*), 5 pieces,
  1.1 oz. 160
peanut butter sandwich (*Nutter Butter*), 2 pieces,
  1 oz. 130
pecan shortbread, see "shortbread," below
raspberry (*Sunshine Oh! Berry*), 3 pieces, 1 oz. 120
raspberry, filled (*Pepperidge Farm Linzer*),
  .8-oz. piece 100
raspberry, filled (*Smart Snackers*), .7 oz. 70
raspberry, hazelnut (*Pepperidge Farm Chantilly*),
  .6-oz. piece 80
shortbread (*Lorna Doone*), 4 pieces, 1 oz. 140
shortbread (*Pepperidge Farm*), 2 pieces, .9 oz. 140
shortbread, fudge striped (*Keebler*), 3 pieces, 1.1 oz. . . . 160
shortbread, fudge striped (*Sunshine*), 3 pieces,
  1.1 oz. 160
shortbread, pecan (*Pecan Sandies*), .6-oz. piece 80
shortbread, pecan (*Pecan Sandies* Reduced Fat),
  .6-oz. piece 70
shortbread, pecan (*Pepperidge Farm*), 2 pieces, .9 oz. . . 140
(*Social Tea*), 6 pieces, 1 oz. 120
spice, pfeffernuss, drops (*Stella D'Oro*), 3 pieces, 1 oz. 120
(*Stella D'Oro Hostess with the Mostest/Lady Stella*
  Assortment), 3 pieces, 1 oz. 130
(*Stella D'Oro Margherite Combination*), 2 pieces,
  1.1 oz. 140
(*Stella D'Oro Royal Nuggets*), 1.1 oz. 140
strawberry (*Pepperidge Farm*), 3 pieces, 1.1 oz. 140
sugar (*Keebler Classic Collection*), 2 pieces, 1 oz. 140
sugar (*Pepperidge Farm*), 3 pieces, 1.1 oz. 140
sugar wafer, chocolate/vanilla (*Sunshine*), 3 pieces,
  .9 oz. 130
sugar wafer, peanut butter (*Sunshine*), 4 pieces, 1.1 oz. 170
vanilla sandwich (*Cameo*), 2 pieces, 1 oz. 130
vanilla sandwich (*Smart Snackers*), 2 pieces, 1.06 oz. . . 140

Cookie *(cont.)*

vanilla sandwich (*SnackWell's* Reduced Fat), 2 pieces,
 .9 oz. 110
vanilla wafer (*Keebler*), 8 pieces, 1.1 oz. 150
vanilla wafer (*Keebler* Light), 8 pieces, 1.1 oz. 130
vanilla wafer (*Nilla*), 8 pieces, 1.1 oz. 140
wafer, fudge (*Keebler Fudge Sticks*), 3 pieces, 1 oz. 150
walnut, black (*Archway* Ice Box), .8-oz. piece 120
wedding cakes (*Archway*), 3 pieces, 1.1 oz. 160

Cookie, refrigerated:

bar, see "Cake, snack, mix"
chocolate chip (*Nestlé/Nestlé* Big Batch), 1 piece* 140
chocolate chip (*Nestlé* Reduced Fat), 1 piece* 130
chocolate chip (*Pillsbury* Reduced Fat), 1 oz. 110
chocolate chip (*SnackWell's*), 1 oz. 110
chocolate chip or chocolate chunk (*Pillsbury*), 1 oz. 130
chocolate chip, oatmeal (*Pillsbury*), 1 oz. 130
chocolate chip, peanut butter (*Nestlé*), 1 piece* 160
chocolate chip, w/walnuts (*Pillsbury*), 1 oz. 140
chocolate chip, chocolate fudge (*SnackWell's*), 1 oz. 90
Heath (*Pillsbury*), 1 oz. 140
M&M's (*Pillsbury*), 1 oz. 130
oatmeal (*Nestlé Scotchies*), 1 piece* 140
peanut butter (*Pillsbury*), 1 oz. 110
Reese's (*Pillsbury*), 1 oz. 130
sugar (*Nestlé*), 1 piece* 120

Cookie crumbs, see "Pie crust"

Cookie mix, 2 pieces*:

chocolate chip (*Duncan Hines*) 170
chocolate chip (*Robin Hood/Gold Medal* Pouch) 170
chocolate chip, oatmeal (*Robin Hood/Gold Medal*
    Pouch) 160
chocolate chunk, double (*Robin Hood/Gold Medal* Pouch) 150
fudge, candy splash (*Duncan Hines*) 140
gingerbread (*Betty Crocker* Fun Kit) 150
peanut butter (*Duncan Hines*) 140
peanut butter (*Robin Hood/Gold Medal* Pouch) 160
sugar (*Duncan Hines*) 150

Cooking sauce, see specific listings

Coquito nut, shelled, (*Frieda's*), 1 oz. 180

Coriander, fresh, ¼ cup 1
Corn, ½ cup, except as noted:
fresh (*Dole*), 1 medium ear, 3.2 oz. 80
fresh, kernels, boiled, drained 89
baby (*Haddon House*) 30
canned, kernel (*Del Monte*) 90
canned, kernel (*Del Monte* Supersweet No Salt/No Sugar) . 60
canned, kernel (*Del Monte* Fiesta) 50
canned, kernel, gold and white (*Del Monte* Supersweet) . 80
canned, kernel, white (*Del Monte*) 80
canned, kernel, w/peppers (*Green Giant Mexicorn*),
   ⅓ cup 60
canned, cream style (*Del Monte/Del Monte* No Salt) . . . 90
canned, cream style (*Del Monte* Supersweet) 60
canned, cream style (*Green Giant*) 100
canned, cream style, white (*Del Monte*) 100
frozen, on the cob (*Birds Eye* Big Ears), 1 ear 120
frozen, on the cob (*Birds Eye* Little Ears), 2 ears 110
frozen, kernel (*Birds Eye*), ⅓ cup 70
frozen, kernel (*Birds Eye* Sweet/Tendersweet), ⅓ cup . . . 60
frozen, kernel, white (*Green Giant*), ¾ cup 100
frozen, kernel, white (*Green Giant* Extra Sweet), ⅔ cup . . 50
frozen, cream style (*Green Giant*) 110
frozen, in butter sauce (*Green Giant Niblets*), ⅔ cup . . . 130
frozen, w/broccoli and peppers (*Green Giant American*
   Mixtures), ¾ cup 60
Corn bread, see "Bread mix"
Corn bread, frozen (*Marie Callender's*), 1.9-oz. piece . . . 150
Corn chips, puffs, and similar snacks:
(*Baked Bugles*), 1½ cups 130
(*Bugles*), 1⅓ cups 160
(*Dipsey Doodles*), 1 oz. 160
(*Fritos* King Size/Original/Wild 'N Mild), 1 oz. 160
(*Fritos* Scoops), 1 oz. 150
all flavors except cheese (*Smart Snackers* Curls), 1 oz. . . 60
all varieties (*Sunchips*), 1 oz. 140
barbecue (*Fritos*), 1 oz. 150
cheese, cheddar (*Baked Bugles*), 1½ cups 130
cheese, nacho (*Bugles*), 1⅓ cups 160
cheese, nacho (*Doodle Twisters*), 1 oz. 160

Corn chips, puffs, and similar snacks *(cont.)*

cheese balls (*Barrel O'Fun*), 1.1 oz. 160
cheese curls (*Barrel O'Fun* Baked/Crunchy), 1.1 oz. 160
cheese curls (*Smart Snackers*), ½ oz. 70
cheese puffs (*Barrel O'Fun* Light), 1.1 oz. 125
cheese puffs (*Jax*), 25 pieces, 1.06 oz. 150
cheese or ranch puffs (*No Fries*), 1 oz. 110
chili cheese (*Fritos*), 1 oz. 160
onion-flavor rings (*Borden*), 1-oz. bag 140
ranch or sour cream and onion (*Bugles*), 1⅓ cups 160
taco (*Taco Bell* Supreme), 1 oz. 140
Texas grill (*Fritos* Honey BBQ/Sizzlin' Fajita), 1 oz. 150
tortilla (*Bachman* Original), 12 pieces, 1.06 oz. 150
tortilla (*Chipitos* Black Bean Salsa), 6 pieces, 1.06 oz. . . 150
tortilla (*Tostitos* Baked/*Tostitos* Baked Unsalted), 1 oz. . . 110
tortilla (*Tostitos* Restaurant), 1 oz. 130
tortilla, all varieties (*Doritos*), 1 oz. 140
tortilla, all varieties (*Doritos* Reduced Fat), 1 oz. 130
tortilla, crisps (*Mr. Phipps*), 1 oz. 130
tortilla, 5 grain or lime and chili (*Kettle* Tias), 1 oz. 140
tortilla, ranch or salsa and sour cream (*No Fries*), 1.1 oz. 110
tortilla, ranch (*Tostitos* Baked), 1 oz. 120
tortilla, blue-corn cheddar jalapeño (*No Fries*), 1.1 oz. . . 110
tortilla, cheese, nacho (*Barrel O'Fun*), 1 oz. 130
tortilla, cheese, nacho, crisps (*Mr. Phipps*), 1 oz. 130
tortilla, flour, yellow (*Barrel O'Fun* Tostada), 1 oz. 130
tortilla, white corn (*Chipitos* Restaurant), 1 oz. 130
tortilla, white corn (*Old El Paso*), 1 oz. 140
tortilla, white corn (*Santitas* 100%), 1 oz. 140
Corn flour:
whole grain, 1 cup 422
masa, 1 cup 416
Corn fritter, frozen (*Mrs. Paul's*), 2 pieces 260
Corn grits, dry, ¼ cup, except as noted:
(*Albers* Quick Hominy) 140
(*Cee-Leci/Dixie Lily/Jim Dandy*) 170
instant, all varieties, except w/ham bits (*Quaker*),
    1-oz. pkt. 100
instant, w/ham bits (*Quaker*), 1-oz. pkt. 90
quick (*Cee-Leci/Dixie Lily/Jim Dandy*) 160

white (*Arrowhead Mills*) 140
yellow (*Dixie Lily/Martha White*) 150
Corn pudding mix (*Goya*), ½ cup* 100
Corn relish (*Green Giant*), 1 tbsp. 20
Corn syrup, dark or light (*Karo*), 2 tbsp. 120
Cornflake crumbs (*Kellogg's*), 2 tbsp. 40
Cornish hen:
roasted, dark meat (*Perdue*), 6.5 oz. 210
roasted, white meat (*Perdue*), 6.5 oz. 200
Cornmeal (see also "Polenta"), 3 tbsp., except as noted:
coarse (*Goya*) 110
fine (*Goya*) 100
masa harina (*Quaker* Enriched), ¼ cup 110
self-rising (*Dixie Lily/Martha White/Pekerson's*) 110
self-rising, buttermilk (*Dixie Lily* Mix) 140
self-rising, white (*Dixie Lily/Mother's Best/Omega*) 140
self-rising, white, plain or honey (*Martha White*) 140
self-rising, yellow, buttermilk (*Martha White* Mix) 150
yellow (*Martha White*) 120
white (*Dixie Lily/Hay Market/Martha White/Pekerson's*) . . 120
white, whole ground (*Cabin Home/Martha White*) 110
Cornstarch (*Argo/Kingsford*), 1 tbsp. 30
Couscous:
dry, regular or whole wheat (*Fantastic Foods*), ¼ cup . . 210
cooked, ½ cup 101
Couscous mix, ⅓ cup:
garlic, w/red pepper (*Fantastic* Healthy Complements) . . 200
pilaf, savory (*Fantastic Foods* Quick) 240
royal Thai (*Fantastic* Healthy Complements) 200
Cowpeas (see also "Black-eyed peas"):
fresh, boiled, drained, ½ cup 79
mature, boiled, ½ cup 100
Crab, meat only, 4 oz.:
Alaska king, boiled, poached, or steamed 110
blue, boiled, poached, or steamed 116
Dungeness, boiled, poached, or steamed 125
queen, boiled, poached, or steamed 130
Crab, refrigerated or frozen:
chunks, cooked (*Tyson* Delight), 3 oz. 70
legs and claws (*Pride of Alaska*), ¾ cup edible 100

Crab, canned, Dungeness (*S&W*), ⅓ cup, 3 oz. 80
"Crab," imitation, frozen or refrigerated:
(*Captain Jac* Easy Shreds), ½ cup 80
flaked (*Captain Jac Crab Tasties*), ½ cup 100
flaked (*Pacific Mate* Fat Free), ½ cup 90
flaked, chunk, or "leg" (*Louis Kemp Crab Delights*), 3 oz.   80
leg style, w/crab (*Captain Jac Crab Tasties*), 3 legs 100
Crab cake, deviled, frozen (*Mrs. Paul's*), 1 piece 170
Crabapple:
fresh, w/peel (*Frieda's*), 1 oz. 19
canned (*S&W*), 1 piece 35
Cracker:
bacon flavor (*Nabisco*), 15 pieces, 1.1 oz. 160
butter or butter flavor:
　(*Goya* Tropical), 4 pieces 140
　(*Hi-Ho*), 9 pieces, 1.1 oz. 160
　(*Keebler Club* Partners), 4 pieces, .5 oz. 70
　(*Ritz*), 5 pieces, .6 oz. 80
　(*Ritz* Low Sodium), 5 pieces, .6 oz. 80
　(*Ritz Air Crisps*), 24 pieces 140
　(*Toasted Complements* Buttercrisp), 9 pieces, 1 oz. . . 140
　(*Town House*), 5 pieces, .6 oz. 80
　mini (*Ritz Bits*), 48 pieces, 1.1 oz. 160
　thins (*Pepperidge Farm*), 4 pieces, .5 oz. 70
cheese:
　(*Krispy* Mild Cheddar), 5 pieces, .5 oz. 60
　(*Nips*), 29 pieces, 1.1 oz. 150
　(*Nips Air Crisps*), 32 pieces 130
　(*SnackWell's*), 38 pieces, 1.1 oz. 130
　(*Tid-Bit*), 32 pieces, 1.1 oz. 150
　cheddar (*Better Cheddars*), 22 pieces, 1.1 oz. 150
　cheddar (*Better Cheddars* Reduced Fat), 24 pieces,
　　1.1 oz. 140
　cheddar (*Cheez-It*), 27 pieces, 1.1 oz. 160
　cheddar (*Cheez-It* Reduced Fat), 30 pieces, 1.1 oz. . . 130
　cheddar (*Combos*), 1 oz. 150
　cheddar (*Munch 'ems*), 30 pieces, 1.1 oz. 130
　cheddar (*Goldfish*), 55 pieces, 1.1 oz. 140
　cheddar, hot and spicy (*Cheez-It*), 26 pieces,
　　1.1 oz. 160

cheddar, white (*Cheez-It*), 26 pieces, 1.1 oz. 160
cheddar, white (*Wheatables*), 27 pieces, 1.1 oz. 130
chili (*Munch 'ems*), 28 pieces, 1.1 oz. 130
Parmesan (*Goldfish*), 60 pieces, 1.1 oz. 140
salsa or zesty (*SnackWell's*), 32 pieces, 1.1 oz. 120
Swiss (*Nabisco Swiss*), 15 pieces, 1 oz. 140
cheese sandwich:
    (*Handi-Snacks* Cheez'n Crackers), 1.1-oz. piece 130
    (*Ritz*), 1.4-oz. pkg. 210
    (*Ritz Bits*), 14 pieces, 1.1 oz. 160
    bacon, jalapeño cheddar, or wheat (*Frito-Lay*),
      1 pkg. 200
    cheddar, golden toast (*Frito-Lay*), 1 pkg. 230
    cream cheese and chive, golden toast (*Frito-Lay*),
      1 pkg. 240
    peanut butter, see "peanut butter," below
(*Chicken In A Biskit*), 14 pieces, 1.1 oz. 160
flatbread:
    all varieties (*J. J. Flats*), .5-oz. piece 50
    all varieties (*New York* Fat Free), .4-oz. piece 40
    plain or Cajun (*New York*), .4-oz. piece 45
    w/everything (*New York*), .4-oz. piece 50
    garlic, onion, or poppy (*California Crisps*), 2 pieces,
      .5 oz. 65
    onion (*New York*), .4-oz. piece 40
    poppy (*New York*), .4-oz. piece 50
    pumpernickel onion (*New York*), .4-oz. piece 40
    pumpernickel sesame (*New York*), .4-oz. piece 50
    sesame (*New York*), .4-oz. piece 50
    10 grain (*California Crisps*), 2 pieces, .5 oz. 59
golden (*SnackWell's* Classic), 6 pieces, .5 oz. 60
(*Goldfish* Original), 55 pieces, 1.1 oz. 140
(*Goya* Snack), 11 pieces 140
(*Goya* Tropical), 4 pieces 140
graham, see "Cookie"
(*Munch'ems*), 30 pieces, 1.1 oz. 130
matzo (*Manischewitz* Unsalted/Everything!), 1 oz. 110
matzo, garlic (*Manischewitz* Savory), 1 oz. 100
matzo, rye (*Manischewitz*), 1 oz. 110

Cracker *(cont.)*

melba rounds, all varieties except garlic and sesame
  (*Devonsheer*), 5 pieces, .5 oz. 50
melba rounds, garlic (*Devonsheer*), 5 pieces, .5 oz. 60
melba rounds, sesame (*Devonsheer*), 5 pieces, .5 oz. . . . 60
melba toast, all varieties (*Devonsheer*), 3 pieces, .5 oz. . . 50
milk (*Royal Lunch*), .4-oz. piece 50
multigrain (*Harvest Crisps*), 13 pieces, 1.1 oz. 130
multigrain (*Wheat Thins*), 17 pieces, 1.1 oz. 130
nori maki (*Eden*), 15 pieces, 1.1 oz. 110
oat (*Harvest Crisps*), 13 pieces, 1.1 oz. 140
oat (*Oat Thins*), 18 pieces, 1.1 oz. 140
onion (*Toasted Complements*), 9 pieces, 1 oz. 140
onion, French (*SnackWell's*), 32 pieces, 1.1 oz. 120
onion, French (*Wheatables*), 29 pieces, 1.1 oz. 130
peanut butter (*Combos*), 1 oz. 140
peanut butter (*Handi-Snacks*), 1.1-oz. piece 180
peanut butter sandwich (*Ritz*), 13 pieces, 1.1 oz. 150
peanut butter sandwich, cheese (*Frito-Lay*), 1 pkg. 200
peanut butter sandwich, cheese (*Nabs*), 6 pieces,
  1.4 oz. 190
peanut butter sandwich, toast (*Frito-Lay*), 1 pkg. 190
peanut butter sandwich, toast (*Nabs*), 6 pieces,
  1.4 oz. 190
pizza (*Goldfish*), 55 pieces, 1.1 oz. 140
potato, all flavors (*No Fries*), 1.1 oz. 110
(*Pretzel Air Crisps*), 22 pieces 110
ranch (*SnackWell's*), 32 pieces 120
ranch (*Wheatables*), 29 pieces, 1.1 oz. 150
rice, brown (*Eden*), 5 pieces, 1.1 oz. 120
saltines (*Premium/Premium* Unsalted), 5 pieces, .5 oz. . . 60
saltines (*Premium* Fat Free), 5 pieces, .5 oz. 50
saltines, mini (*Premium* Bits), 34 pieces, 1.1 oz. 150
sesame (*Pepperidge Farm*), 3 pieces, .5 oz. 70
sesame (*Toasted Complements*), 10 pieces, 1 oz. 140
sesame cheese (*Twigs*), 15 pieces, 1.1 oz. 150
(*Sociables*), 7 pieces, .5 oz. 80
soup and oyster (*Krispy*), .5 oz. 60
(*Uneeda*), 2 pieces, .5 oz. 60
vegetable (*Garden Crisps*), 15 pieces, 1.1 oz. 130

vegetable (*Vegetable Thins*), 14 pieces, 1.1 oz. 160
water or soda:
   (*Carr's Table Water*), 5 pieces, .6 oz. 70
   (*Crown Pilot*), .6-oz. piece 70
   (*Dux*), 2 pieces 40
   (*Pepperidge Farm*), 5 pieces, .5 oz. 60
   cracked pepper (*Carr's Table Water*), 5 pieces, .6 oz. . . 70
   cracked pepper (*Pepperidge Farm*), 5 pieces, .5 oz. . . . 60
   cracked pepper (*SnackWell's*), 7 pieces, .5 oz. 60
   poppy sesame (*Carr's*), 4 pieces, .5 oz. 80
   sesame (*Carr's Table Water*), 5 pieces, .6 oz. 70
wheat:
   (*SnackWell's* Fat Free), 5 pieces, .5 oz. 60
   (*Stoned Wheat Thins*), 2 pieces 60
   (*Toasted Complements*), 9 pieces, 1 oz. 140
   (*Triscuit*), 7 pieces, 1.1 oz. 140
   (*Triscuit* Low Sodium), 7 pieces, 1.1 oz. 150
   (*Triscuit* Reduced Fat), 8 pieces, 1.1 oz. 130
   (*Waverly*), 5 pieces, .5 oz. 70
   (*Wheat Thins*), 16 pieces, 1 oz. 140
   (*Wheat Thins* Reduced Fat), 18 pieces, 1 oz. 120
   (*Wheat Thins Air Crisps*), 24 pieces 130
   (*Wheatables*), 26 pieces, 1.1 oz. 150
   (*Wheatsworth*), 5 pieces, .6 oz. 80
   cracked (*Pepperidge Farm*), 2 pieces, .5 oz. 70
   hearty (*Pepperidge Farm*), 3 pieces, .5 oz. 80
   herb, garden (*Triscuit*), 6 pieces, 1 oz. 130
   whole (*Carr's*), 2 pieces, .6 oz. 80
   whole, and bran (*Triscuit*), 7 pieces, 1.1 oz. 140
wheat and rye (*Triscuit* Deli), 7 pieces, 1.1 oz. 140
(*Zwieback*), .3-oz. piece 35
Cracker crumbs and meal:
crumbs (*Ritz*), 1/3 cup 140
crumbs, saltine (*Premium* Fat Free), 1/4 cup 100
matzo meal (*Streit's*), 1/4 cup 110
Cranberry, fresh, raw, whole (*Dole*), 1/2 cup 23
Cranberry, dried (*Craisins*), 1/3 cup 130
Cranberry bean, canned, w/liquid, 1/2 cup 108
Cranberry drink:
(*Farmer's Market*), 8 fl. oz. 120

juice cocktail (*Seneca*), 8 fl. oz. 140
frozen, juice cocktail (*Seneca*), 2 oz. 140
Cranberry drink blends, 8 fl. oz.:
hibiscus (*Heinke's*). 120
lemon (*Santa Cruz*) 120
raspberry (*After the Fall*) 90
raspberry-strawberry (*Tropicana Twister*) 120
raspberry-strawberry (*Tropicana Twister* Light) 45
Cranberry juice:
(*R. W. Knudsen* Just Cranberry), 8 fl. oz. 60
(*R. W. Knudsen* Yankee), 8 fl. oz. 120
(*Ocean Spray* Cocktail), 6 fl. oz. 100
Cranberry juice blend, 8 fl. oz.:
apple (*Cranapple*) 160
blueberry (*Cran·Blueberry*) 160
grape (*Cran·Grape*) 170
grapefruit or orange (*After the Fall*) 110
kiwi, mango, or strawberry (*After the Fall*) 100
punch (*Crantastic*) 150
raspberry (*After the Fall*) 90
strawberry (*Ocean Spray*) 140
Cranberry nectar (*R. W. Knudsen*), 8 fl. oz. 150
Cranberry sauce, whole or jellied (*Ocean Spray*), 2 oz. . . 80
Cranberry sauce blends, all varieties (*Cran·Fruit*), 2 oz. . . 90
Cranberry-orange relish, in jars (*New England*),
  1/4 cup 120
Crayfish, mixed species, meat only, 4 oz.:
wild, boiled or steamed 100
farmed, boiled or steamed 99
Cream, dairy pack:
half-and-half (*Breakstone's*), 2 tbsp. 45
light, coffee or table, 1 tbsp. 29
medium (25% fat), 1 tbsp. 37
sour, see "Cream, sour"
whipping[1], light, 1 tbsp. 44
whipping[1], heavy (*America's Choice*), 1 tbsp. 50
whipped topping, see "Cream topping"
Cream, canned, light (*Nestlé* Crema), 1 tbsp. 30

---

[1] *Unwhipped; volume approximately doubled when whipped.*

Cream, sour, 2 tbsp.:
(*Land O Lakes*) 60
(*Land O Lakes* Light) 35
(*Land O Lakes* No Fat) 30
nondairy, plain or flavored (*Sour Supreme*) 50
Cream of tartar (*Tone's*), 1 tsp. 2
Cream topping, 2 tbsp.:
(*Kraft* Real) 20
(*Kraft* Whipped Topping) 20
(*La Crema* Lite) 15
pressurized can (*Rich's*) 25
Cream topping mix (*D-Zerta*), 2 tbsp.* 10
Creamer, nondairy:
(*Coffee-mate*), 1 tbsp. 20
(*Coffee-mate* Fat Free), 1 tbsp. 10
(*Coffee-mate* Lite), 1 tbsp. 10
powder (*Coffee-mate/Coffee-mate* Lite), 1 tsp. 10
flavored, all flavors, liquid (*Coffee-mate*), 1 tbsp. 40
flavored, all flavors, powder (*Coffee-mate*), 1 1/3 tbsp. 60
Crepe, fresh (*Frieda's*), 1 piece 45
Cress, garden, raw, 1/2 cup 8
Croaker, meat only, raw, Atlantic, 4 oz. 119
Croissant:
butter (*Pepperidge Farm* Petite), 1 piece 130
frozen (*Sara Lee* Original), 1 piece 170
frozen, petite (*Sara Lee*), 2 pieces 230
Crookneck squash, 1/2 cup:
fresh, boiled, drained, sliced 18
canned, cut, yellow (*Allens/Sunshine*) 16
frozen, boiled, drained, sliced 24
Croutons:
Caesar, cheese/garlic, cracked pepper/Parmesan, ranch,
  seasoned, or zesty Italian (*Pepperidge Farm*),
  2 tbsp. 35
Caesar (*Pepperidge Farm* Fat Free), 6 pieces, .3 oz. 30
cheddar/Romano, olive oil/garlic, onion/garlic, or cheese
  sourdough (*Pepperidge Farm*), 2 tbsp. 30
Italian, spicy (*Pepperidge Farm* Fat Free), 6 pieces,
  .3 oz. 30

Cucumber, w/peel:

(*Dole*), ⅓ medium 15

hothouse (*Frieda's*), 1 oz. 4

Cucumber dip, creamy (*Kraft* Premium), 2 tbsp. 50

Cucumber salad (*Rosoff/Schorr's*), 1 oz. 12

Cumin seed, ground (*McCormick*), ¼ tsp. 3

Cupcake, see "Cake, snack" and "Cake, snack, mix"

Currant, trimmed:

fresh, black, European, ½ cup 36

fresh, red or white, ½ cup 31

dried, Zante (*S&W*), ¼ cup 130

Curry paste (*Patak's*), 2 tbsp. 170

Curry powder (*Tone's*), ¼ tsp. 0

Curry sauce mix (*Knorr*), ⅕ pkg. 30

Cusk, meat only, baked, broiled, or microwaved, 4 oz. . . 127

Custard apple, trimmed, 1 oz. 29

Cuttlefish, meat only, boiled or steamed, 4 oz. 179

Cuttlefish, canned, in ink (*Goya*), ¼ cup 120

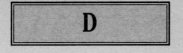

D

FOOD AND MEASURE   **CALORIES**

Daiquiri mixer:
bottled (*Holland House/Mr & Mrs T*), 4 fl. oz. 150
frozen*, banana (*Bacardi*), 8 fl. oz. 140
frozen*, strawberry or peach (*Bacardi*), 8 fl. oz. 120
mix (*Bar-Tenders*), 2 pkts., 1.2 oz. 30
Dandelion greens, boiled, drained, chopped, ½ cup 17
Danish, frozen, 1 piece:
apple or raspberry (*Pepperidge Farm*) 210
cheese (*Pepperidge Farm*) 230
Date:
dehydrated, fine or coarse ground (*Dole*), 1 oz. 110
dried, pitted (*Del Monte*), 5–6 pieces, 1.4 oz. 120
dried, pitted, chopped (*Del Monte*), 1.4 oz., ¼ cup 120
Date nut loaf, see "Bread mix, sweet"
Demiglace sauce mix (*Knorr*), 1 tbsp. 30
Denny's, 1 serving:
breakfast, w/out bread:
    All American Slam 1,028
    Belgian waffle, plain 304
    Belgian waffle supreme, w/out bacon or sausage . . . 433
    chicken-fried steak and eggs 723
    French Slam 1,029
    French toast, plain, 2 pieces 510
    ham 'n' cheddar omelette 743
    Moons Over My Hammy, w/out potato 807
    Original *Grand Slam,* w/out syrup, margarine 795
    pancakes, plain, 3 pieces 491
    pork chop and eggs 555
    porterhouse steak and eggs 1,223
    Scram Slam 974
    Senior Belgian Waffle Slam, w/out syrup, margarine 399
    Senior Omelette 623
    Senior Starter, w/out bacon or sausage 336

Denny's, breakfast, w/out bread *(cont.)*

Senior Triple Play, w/out bacon or sausage 537
sirloin steak and eggs 808
Slim Slam, w/syrup, w/out topping 638
Southern Slam 1,065
Super/Play It Again Slam 1,192
T-bone steak and eggs 1,045
Ultimate Omelette 780
veggie-cheese omelette 714

breakfast, junior:

basic breakfast 558
Belgian waffle 190
Junior French Slam, w/out syrup, margarine 461
Junior Grand Slam, w/out syrup, margarine 397

breakfast items:

apple juice, 10 oz. 126
applesauce 60
bacon, 4 slices 162
bagel, dry, whole 235
banana 110
banana/strawberry medley 108
biscuit, plain 375
biscuit and sausage gravy 570
cantaloupe, 3 oz. 32
cereal, dry, average, 1 oz. 100
cream cheese, 1 oz. 100
egg, 1 134
egg substitute, Sunny Fresh 94
grapefruit, 1/2 60
grapefruit juice, 10 oz. 115
grapes, 3 oz. 55
grits, 4 oz. 80
ham, 3 oz. 94
hashed browns 218
hashed browns, covered 318
hashed browns, covered and smothered 359
honeydew 31
margarine, whipped, .5 oz. 87
muffin, blueberry 309
muffin, English, plain, dry 125

oatmeal, 4 oz. 100
orange juice, 10 oz. 126
sausage, 4 links 354
strawberries, frozen, w/sugar, 3 oz. 115
syrup, 1.5 oz. 143
syrup, reduced calorie, 1.5 oz. 25
toast, dry, 1 slice 92
tomato juice, 10 oz. 56
topping, blueberry, 3 oz. 106
topping, strawberry, 3 oz. 115
salad, w/out dressing, except as noted:
  fried chicken 506
  garden chicken delite 119
  grilled chicken Caesar, w/dressing 655
  Oriental chicken, w/dressing 568
  side Caesar, w/dressing 338
  side garden 113
dressings, 1 oz.:
  bleu cheese 124
  Caesar 142
  French 106
  French, reduced calorie 76
  honey mustard, fat free 38
  Italian, creamy 106
  Italian, reduced calorie 23
  Oriental 106
  ranch 101
  Thousand Island 104
condiments, 1.5 oz.:
  BBQ sauce 47
  horseradish sauce 170
  sour cream 91
soup, 8 oz.:
  cheese 293
  chicken noodle 60
  clam chowder 214
  cream of broccoli 193
  cream of potato 222
  split pea 146
  vegetable beef 79

Denny's (cont.)

sandwiches, w/out fries or substitutes:

bacon Swiss burger	710
bacon, lettuce, and tomato	634
Charleston Chicken	566
chicken melt	520
club	718
Delidinger	852
deluxe grilled cheese	482
Denny Burger	513
French dip, w/out horseradish sauce	531
fried fish	905
grilled chicken	436
Humdinger Hamburger	748
patty melt	694
Super Bird	620

sandwiches, lunch combinations:

ham and Swiss on rye, w/out soup, salad	533
turkey breast on multigrain, w/out soup, salad	476

sandwiches, senior, sandwich only:

half grilled cheese	246
ham and Swiss, w/out fries or substitutes	497
turkey, w/out fries or substitutes	476

appetizers, w/out condiments, except as noted:

Buffalo chicken strips	734
Buffalo wings, 12 pieces	856
chicken quesadilla	827
chicken strips, 5 pieces	720
mozzarella sticks, 8 pieces, w/sauce	756
onion rings, 7 pieces	439
Sampler	1,120

entrees [1]:

battered cod, w/tartar sauce	732
Charleston Chicken	327
chicken-fried steak	265
chicken strip, w/honey mustard dressing	635
Denny Cut prime rib, 8 oz., w/au jus and horseradish	760

[1] Add bread; choice of salad, soup, or fruit; choice of potato or rice pilaf; and choice of vegetable.

grilled Alaskan salmon 296
grilled breast of chicken 130
liver w/bacon and onions 497
pork chop dinner 386
porterhouse steak 708
roast turkey and stuffing 701
shrimp 558
steak and shrimp 645
T-bone steak dinner 530
junior meals, w/out fries or substitutes:
  burger 261
  fried fish 465
  grilled cheese 375
  shrimp basket 291
senior meals [1]:
  battered cod, w/out potato or pilaf 465
  chicken-fried steak 341
  grilled chicken breast 219
  liver w/bacon and onions 322
  pork chop 193
  pot roast 149
  turkey and stuffing 596
sides:
  broccoli in butter sauce, 4 oz. 50
  carrots in honey glaze, 4 oz. 80
  corn in butter sauce, 4 oz. 120
  corn bread stuffing, 2 oz. 182
  french fries, unsalted, 4 oz. 323
  fries, seasoned, 4 oz. 261
  gravy, brown, 1 oz. 13
  gravy, chicken, 1 oz. 14
  gravy, country, 1 oz. 17
  green beans w/bacon, 4 oz. 60
  green peas in butter sauce, 4 oz. 100
  potato, baked, plain, 6 oz. 186
  potato, mashed, plain, 6 oz. 105
  rice pilaf, 3 oz. 112
  sliced tomatoes, 3 slices 13

[1] *Add bread; choice of soup, salad, or fruit; and choice of vegetable.*

Denny's (cont.)
pies, "Mother Butler," ⅙ pie:
 apple 430
 apple, w/*Equal* 370
 cherry 540
 chocolate pecan 790
 coconut cream 480
 cheesecake pie 470
 Dutch apple 440
 French silk 650
 German chocolate 580
 key lime or pecan 600
 lemon meringue 460
other desserts:
 banana split sundae, 19 oz. 894
 chocolate cake, 4 oz. 370
 hot fudge cake sundae, 8 oz. 687
 sundae, double scoop, 6 oz., w/out topping 375
 sundae, single scoop, 3 oz., w/out topping 188
 tapioca, 4 oz. 127
dessert toppings:
 blueberry, 2 oz. 71
 cheesecake, blueberry, 3 oz. 106
 cheesecake, cherry, 3 oz. 115
 chocolate, 2 oz. 317
 fudge, 2 oz. 201
 strawberry, 2 oz. 77
coffee, French vanilla, 8 oz. 76
coffee, hazelnut, 8 oz. 66
coffee, Irish cream, 8 oz. 73
Dessert filling, see "Pie filling"
Dessert mix, chilled, no-bake:
banana cream (*Betty Crocker*), ⅑ dessert* 250
chocolate French silk (*Betty Crocker*), ⅛ dessert* 270
coconut cream (*Betty Crocker*), ⅑ dessert* 290
cookies 'n creme (*Betty Crocker*), ⅙ dessert* 360
Sunkist lemon supreme (*Betty Crocker*), ⅑ dessert* . . . 320
Diable sauce (*Escoffier*), 1 tbsp. 20
Dill:
fresh, 5 sprigs . . . . <1

dried, seed (*McCormick*), ¼ tsp. 3
dried, weed (*McCormick*), ¼ tsp. 1
Dill dip, 2 tbsp.:
(*Bernstein's* Zesty) 120
(*Heluva* Good) 60
Dock, boiled, drained, 4 oz. 23
Dolphinfish, meat only, 4 oz.:
raw 97
baked, broiled, or microwaved 124
frozen, fillet (*Peter Pan* Mahi Mahi) 100
Domino's Pizza:
cheese pizza, 12″ medium pie:
  deep dish, 2 of 8 slices 467
  hand-tossed, 2 of 8 slices 349
  thin crust, ¼ pie 273
  "Add a Topping" anchovies 23
  "Add a Topping" bacon 82
  "Add a Topping" beef, precooked 56
  "Add a Topping" cheddar cheese 57
  "Add a Topping" extra cheese 49
  "Add a Topping" ham 18
  "Add a Topping" mushrooms, fresh or canned 4
  "Add a Topping" olives, green 12
  "Add a Topping" olives, ripe 14
  "Add a Topping" onion 4
  "Add a Topping" pepperoni 62
  "Add a Topping" peppers, banana or green 3
  "Add a Topping" pineapple tidbits 10
  "Add a Topping" sausage, Italian 55
cheese pizza, 14″ large pie:
  deep dish, 2 of 12 slices 464
  hand-tossed, 2 of 12 slices 319
  thin crust, ⅙ pie 255
  "Add a Topping" anchovies 23
  "Add a Topping" bacon 75
  "Add a Topping" beef, precooked 44
  "Add a Topping" cheddar cheese 48
  "Add a Topping" extra cheese 46
  "Add a Topping" ham 17
  "Add a Topping" mushrooms, fresh or canned 3

Domino's Pizza, cheese pizza, 14″ large pie *(cont.)*
"Add a Topping" olives, green 11
"Add a Topping" olives, ripe 12
"Add a Topping" onion 3
"Add a Topping" pepperoni 55
"Add a Topping" peppers, banana 3
"Add a Topping" peppers, green 2
"Add a Topping" pineapple tidbits 8
"Add a Topping" sausage, Italian 44
cheese pizza, 6″ deep dish, 1 pie:
plain 591
"Add a Topping" anchovies 45
"Add a Topping" bacon 82
"Add a Topping" beef, precooked 44
"Add a Topping" cheddar cheese 86
"Add a Topping" extra cheese 59
"Add a Topping" ham 17
"Add a Topping" mushrooms, fresh or canned 2
"Add a Topping" olives, green 10
"Add a Topping" olives, ripe 11
"Add a Topping" onion 3
"Add a Topping" pepperoni 50
"Add a Topping" peppers, banana 3
"Add a Topping" peppers, green 2
"Add a Topping" pineapple tidbits 5
"Add a Topping" sausage, Italian 44
Buffalo wings, barbecue, 1 piece 50
Buffalo wings, hot, 1 piece 45
breadstick, 1 piece 78
cheesy bread, 1 piece 103
salad, small 22
salad, large 39
Marzetti salad dressings, 1.5 oz.:
blue cheese 220
Caesar, creamy 200
French, honey 210
Italian, house 220
Italian, light 20
ranch 260

ranch, fat free 40
Thousand Island 200
Donut, 1 piece, except as noted:
plain (*Hostess*) 140
blueberry (*Hostess*) 210
cinnamon sugar (*Entenmann's* Variety Pack) 310
crumb (*Entenmann's*) 260
crumb (*Entenmann's* Variety Pack) 420
crumb (*Hostess Donettes*), 6 pieces, 3 oz. 320
crumb, devil's food (*Entenmann's*) 250
chocolate iced (*Hostess*) 180
chocolate iced (*Hostess Donettes*), 6 pieces, 3 oz. 390
chocolate iced, mini (*Entenmann's*), 2 pieces 270
chocolate iced, rich (*Entenmann's*) 280
chocolate iced, rich (*Entenmann's* Variety Pack) 400
chocolate iced, rich, mini (*Entenmann's Popettes*),
    3 pieces 210
chocolate iced, rich, w/raspberry (*Entenmann's*) 260
glazed (*Entenmann's Popems*), 6 pieces 240
glazed (*Hostess*) 270
glazed, buttermilk (*Entenmann's*) 270
glazed, chocolate (*Entenmann's Popems*), 4 pieces 200
powdered sugar (*Entenmann's*) 220
powdered sugar (*Hostess Donettes*), 6 pieces, 3 oz. . . . 350
powdered sugar, cinnamon (*Hostess*) 150
raspberry filled (*Hostess O's*) 230
stick, see "Cake, snack"
Donut, frozen, glazed (*Rich's*), 1 piece 130
Drum, freshwater, meat only, 4 oz.:
raw 135
baked, broiled, or microwaved 173
Duck, domesticated, 4 oz.:
roasted, meat w/skin 382
roasted, meat only 228
Duck sauce, see "Sweet and sour sauce"
Dumpling entree, frozen, Oriental (*Lean Cuisine*), 9 oz.   320

E

Eclair, chocolate, frozen, 1 piece:
(*Weight Watchers*) 150
triple (*Weight Watchers*) 160
Eel, meat only, 4 oz.:
raw 209
baked, broiled, or microwaved 268
Egg, chicken:
raw, whole, 1 large 75
raw, white only, from 1 large egg 17
raw, yolk (w/small portion white), from 1 large egg 59
cooked, poached, 1 large 74
Egg, substitute or imitation, 1/4 cup:
(*Egg Watchers*) 30
(*Morningstar Farms Better'n Eggs*) 20
(*Morningstar Farms Scramblers*) 35
Egg breakfast, frozen (see also specific listings), 1 pkg.:
omelet, ham and cheese (*Weight Watchers*) 220
scrambled, and bacon (*Swanson Great Starts*) 290
scrambled, w/Canadian bacon (*Swanson Great Starts*
   Low Fat/Cholesterol) 240
scrambled, w/home fries (*Swanson Great Starts*) 200
scrambled, and pancake (*Swanson Great Starts* Low Fat/
   Cholesterol) 220
scrambled, and sausage (*Swanson Great Starts*) 360
scrambled, w/sausage and home fries (*Swanson Great
   Starts* Low Fat/Cholesterol) 240
Egg breakfast sandwich, frozen, 1 pkg.:
biscuit, see "Sausage biscuit"
w/cheese (*Swanson Great Starts*) 350
muffin (*Weight Watchers*) 210
muffin, w/bacon and cheese (*Swanson Great Starts*) . . . 290
omelet (*Weight Watchers* Classic) 220

Egg roll, frozen:

(*Empire* Kosher Mini), 6 rolls 280

chicken or pork (*Chun King/La Choy*), 3-oz. roll 170

chicken, mini (*Chun King*), 12 rolls 400

shrimp (*Chun King/La Choy*), 3-oz. roll 150

shrimp or pork and shrimp, mini (*Chun King*), 12 rolls . . 420

Egg roll entree, frozen, vegetable (*Lean Cuisine*), 9 oz.   330

Egg roll wrapper (*Nasoya*), 1.5 oz. 117

Eggnog, dairy, ½ cup:

(*Borden*) 160

(*Borden* Light) 150

Eggplant, fresh:

raw, trimmed, 1″ pieces, ½ cup 11

boiled, drained, 1″ cubes, ½ cup 13

Japanese, raw, w/peel (*Frieda's*), 3½ oz. 25

Eggplant appetizer:

(*Progresso* Caponata), 2 tbsp. 25

stuffed, baby (*Krinos*), 1.1 oz., approx. 2 pieces 20

stuffed, rolettes (*Paesana*), 3¾ oz. 260

Eggplant dip (*Victoria*), 2 tbsp. 30

Eggplant entree, frozen:

cutlets (*Celentano*), 5 oz. 210

parmigiana (*Celentano*), 10-oz. pkg. 420

parmigiana (*Mrs. Paul's*), ½ cup 220

rollettes (*Celentano*), 10 oz. 350

Elderberry, fresh, ½ cup 53

Enchilada dinner, frozen, 1 pkg., except as noted:

(*Amy's*), 10 oz. 250

(*Chi-Chi's* Baja), 15.4 oz. 580

beef (*Patio*), 12 oz. 350

beef (*Swanson*) 470

beef, w/chili sauce (*Banquet* Family), 4.7-oz. piece 130

cheese (*Patio*), 12 oz. 330

chicken (*Chi-Chi's* Suprema), 14.9 oz. 580

chicken (*Healthy Choice* Suprema), 11.3 oz. 270

chicken (*Patio*), 12 oz. 380

Enchilada entree, frozen:

beef or beef and cheese (*Patio* Chili 'n Beans Large),

2 pieces, 7¾ oz. 250

black bean (*Amy's* Family), 4.38 oz. 120

Enchilada entree *(cont.)*
black bean and vegetable (*Amy's* Family), 4.75 oz. 130
cheese (*Amy's*), 4.75 oz. 210
cheese and rice (*Stouffer's*), 9¾ oz. 370
chicken (*Stouffer's* 57 oz.), 4.75 oz. 230
chicken and rice (*Stouffer's*), 10 oz. 370
chicken Suiza (*Healthy Choice*), 10 oz. 270
chicken Suiza (*Weight Watchers*), 9 oz. 270
chicken Suiza, w/rice (*Lean Cuisine*), 9 oz. 280
Enchilada sauce, ¼ cup:
(*Rosarita*) 25
all varieties (*Old El Paso*) 30
original or hot (*Las Palmas*) 15
green chili (*Las Palmas*) 25
Enchilada seasoning mix (*Old El Paso*), 2 tsp. 10
Endive, chopped, ½ cup 4
Endive, Belgian, see "Chicory, witloof"
Escarole, see "Endive"

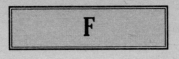

F

FOOD AND MEASURE   **CALORIES**

Fajita, canned, beef or chicken (*Nalley* Superba), 1 cup   230
Fajita mix (*Old El Paso*), 2 pieces* 330
Fajita sauce, marinade (*World Harbors* Guadalupe),
   2 tbsp. 50
Fajita seasoning mix (*Old El Paso*), 1 tbsp. 30
Falafel mix (*Casbah*), ⅛ pkg. 130
Farina, whole grain (see also "Cereal"):
dry, 1 oz. 105
cooked, 1 cup 116
Fat, see specific listings
Fat, imitation (*Rokeach Nyafat*), 1 tbsp. 99
Fava beans, see "Broad beans"
Feijoa, raw:
pureed, ½ cup 60
(*Frieda's*), 1 oz. 17
Fennel, bulb, raw, trimmed, 1 bulb, 8.3 oz. 72
Fennel seed, 1 tsp. 7
Fettuccine, plain:
dry, see "Pasta"
refrigerated, plain or spinach (*Di Giorno*), 2.5 oz. 190
Fettuccine entree, frozen:
Alfredo (*Lean Cuisine*), 9 oz. 300
Alfredo (*Stouffer's*), 10 oz. 520
Alfredo, w/four cheeses (*The Budget Gourmet* Special
   Selections), 11.5 oz. 480
chicken, see "Chicken entree"
and meatballs, in wine sauce (*The Budget Gourmet*
   Italian Originals), 10¼ oz. 320
primavera (*Lean Cuisine*), 9 oz. 280
primavera (*Stouffer's*), 10 oz. 430
primavera, in herb sauce, w/chicken (*The Budget
   Gourmet* Italian Originals), 10 oz. 270

Fettuccine entree mix, approx. 1 cup*:

w/Alfredo sauce (*Pasta Roni*) 470

broccoli, au gratin (*Pasta Roni*) 280

cheddar, mild (*Pasta Roni*) 290

chicken sauce (*Pasta Roni*) 320

Romanoff (*Pasta Roni*) 400

Fig:

fresh, California, 4 figs, 2 oz. 143

fresh, Calimyrna (*Frieda's*), 1 oz. 23

canned, in syrup, Kadota (*S&W*), 5 figs 140

dried, Calamata string (*Agora*), ½ cup 250

dried, white or mission (*Sonoma*), 3–4 figs, 1.4 oz. 110

Filbert:

dried, 1 oz. 179

dry-roasted, salted or unsalted, 1 oz. 188

oil-roasted, salted or unsalted, 1 oz. 187

Fillo pastry, frozen (*Apollo*), ⅛ pkg. 180

Finnan haddie, see "Haddock, smoked"

Fish, see specific listings

"Fish," vegetarian:

frozen (*Worthington*), 2 fillets 180

mix (*Loma Linda* Ocean Platter), ⅓ cup 90

Fish batter mix, see "Fish seasoning and coating mix"

Fish dinner, frozen (see also specific fish listings):

baked, herb (*Healthy Choice*), 10.9 oz. 340

lemon pepper (*Healthy Choice*), 10.7 oz. 290

Fish entree, frozen (see also specific fish listings):

fillet, baked (*Van de Kamp's* Crisp & Healthy), 2 pieces 150

fillet, baked, garlic and pepper (*Mrs. Paul's*), 1 piece . . . 150

fillet, baked, garlic and pepper (*Van de Kamp's*), 1 piece 150

fillet, baked, lemon pepper (*Mrs. Paul's*), 1 piece 140

fillet, baked, lemon pepper (*Van de Kamp's*), 1 piece . . . 140

fillet, battered (*Mrs. Paul's*), 1 piece 170

fillet, battered (*Van de Kamp's*), 1 piece 180

fillet, breaded (*Mrs. Paul's* Crisp & Healthy), 2 fillets . . . 150

fillet, breaded (*Van de Kamp's*), 2 pieces 280

fillet, breaded, cornmeal (*Mrs. Paul's*), 1 piece 180

fillet, breaded, cornmeal (*Van de Kamp's*), 1 piece 180

fillet, grilled, all varieties (*Mrs. Paul's*), 1 piece 130

fillet, grilled, all varieties (*Van de Kamp's*), 1 piece 130

fillet, in butter-flavored sauce (*Mrs. Paul's*), 1 piece . . . 120
w/macaroni and cheese (*Stouffer's* Homestyle), 9 oz. . . . 430
nuggets (*Van de Kamp's*), 8 pieces 280
portions, battered (*Van de Kamp's*), 2 pieces 350
portions, breaded (*Van de Kamp's*), 3 pieces 330
sticks, battered (*Van de Kamp's*), 6 pieces 260
sticks, breaded (*Mrs. Paul's*), 6 pieces 200
sticks, breaded (*Mrs. Paul's* Crisp & Healthy), 6 pieces 180
sticks, breaded, mini (*Van de Kamp's*), 13 pieces 250
Fish sandwich, fillet, frozen, 1 piece:
(*Hormel Quick Meal*) 400
w/cheese (*Mrs. Paul's*) 330
Fish sauce mix, lemon butter (*Weight Watchers*),
   1/4 cup* 5
Fish seasoning, seafood (*Tone's*), 1 tsp. 10
Fish seasoning and coating mix:
lemon pepper dill (*Durkee Easy*), 1/6 pkg. 20
tomato basil (*Durkee Easy*), 1/7 pkg. 15
Flatbread, see "Cracker"
Flatfish, meat only, 4 oz.:
raw 104
baked, broiled, or microwaved 133
Flavor enhancer (*Ac'cent*), 1/2 tsp. 5
Flounder, frozen (*Van de Kamp's*), 4 oz. 110
Flounder entree, fillets, frozen:
breaded (*Van de Kamp's* Light), 3.98-oz. piece 230
Flour, see "Wheat flour" and other specific listings
Fra diavolo sauce, see "Pasta sauce"
Frankfurter, 1 link, except as noted:
(*John Morrell* Fat Free), 1.4 oz. 45
(*John Morrell* Lite) 90
(*Louis Rich* Wieners) 70
(*Oscar Mayer* Wieners) 150
(*Oscar Mayer* Wieners Light) 110
beef (*Hebrew National*), 1.7 oz. 150
beef (*Louis Rich*) 70
beef (*Oscar Mayer*) 140
cheese (*Oscar Mayer*) 140
cocktail, beef (*Boar's Head*), 5 links 170
smoked (*Oscar Mayer Big & Juicy* Smokie) 220

Turkey, see "Turkey frankfurter"
"Frankfurter," vegetarian, 1 link:
(*NewMenu* VegiDog) 45
canned (*Loma Linda* Big) 110
frozen, corn battered (*Loma Linda* Corn Dog) 220
refrigerated, chili (*Yves Veggie Cuisine* Dogs) 70
refrigerated, tofu (*Yves Veggie Cuisine* Wieners) 57
Franks and beans, see "Beans and franks"
French toast, frozen, plain or cinnamon swirl (*Aunt
    Jemima*), 2 pieces 240
French toast breakfast, frozen, 1 pkg.:
cinnamon swirl (*Swanson Great Starts*) 440
w/sausage (*Swanson Great Starts*) 410
Frosting, ready-to-spread, 2 tbsp., except as noted:
all flavors, except chocolate (*Betty Crocker* Whipped
    Deluxe) 110
all flavors except chocolate (*Duncan Hines*) 130
butter cream or pecan (*Betty Crocker Creamy Deluxe*) . . 150
caramel chocolate chip (*Betty Crocker Creamy Deluxe*) . . 140
cherry (*Betty Crocker Creamy Deluxe*) 140
chocolate, all chocolate flavors (*Duncan Hine*) 140
chocolate or milk chocolate:
    (*Betty Crocker* Sweet Rewards), 1 tbsp. 130
    (*Betty Crocker* Whipped Deluxe) 100
    (*Betty Crocker Creamy Deluxe* Low Fat) 120
    or dark chocolate (*Betty Crocker Creamy Deluxe*) . . . 150
chocolate, sour cream, or Swiss almond (*Betty Crocker
    Creamy Deluxe*) 150
chocolate chip (*Betty Crocker Creamy Deluxe*) 160
chocolate chip cookie dough (*Betty Crocker Creamy
    Deluxe*) 160
chocolate chocolate chip (*Betty Crocker Creamy Deluxe*) 150
chocolate fudge or milk chocolate (*SnackWell's*) 120
coconut pecan (*Betty Crocker Creamy Deluxe*) 150
cream cheese (*Betty Crocker Creamy Deluxe*) 140
lemon (*Betty Crocker Creamy Deluxe*) 140
rainbow chip (*Betty Crocker Creamy Deluxe*) 160
strawberry, cream cheese (*Betty Crocker Creamy Deluxe*) 150
vanilla (*Betty Crocker Creamy Deluxe* Low Fat) 120
vanilla (*Betty Crocker* Sweet Rewards), 1 tbsp. 130

vanilla (*SnackWell's*) 130
vanilla or white chocolate (*Betty Crocker Creamy Deluxe*) 140
white, sour cream (*Betty Crocker Creamy Deluxe*) 150
Frosting mix, 2 tbsp.*:
chocolate (*Robin Hood*) 140
chocolate fudge (*Betty Crocker*) 140
coconut pecan (*Betty Crocker*) 160
vanilla (*Betty Crocker*) 130
Fructose (*Estee*), 1 tsp. 16
Fruit, see specific listings
Fruit, mixed, candied (see also specific listings):
(*White Swan*), 1 tbsp., .8 oz. 70
(*White Swan* Deluxe), 2 tbsp., 1.2 oz. 100
Fruit, mixed, canned or in jars (see also "Fruit
    cocktail"):
in juice, chunky (*S&W* Natural), ½ cup 70
in juice or light syrup (*Del Monte* Naturals Snack Cup),
    4-oz. cup 50
in extra light syrup, chunky (*Del Monte* Lite), ½ cup 60
in heavy syrup (*Del Monte* Snack Cup), 4-oz. cup 80
salad, in light syrup (*Sunfresh/Sunfresh* Ambrosia),
    ½ cup 70
salad, tropical, in light syrup (*Sunfresh*), ½ cup 80
Fruit, mixed, dried:
(*Del Monte*), ⅓ cup, 1.4 oz. 110
and nuts, see "Trail mix"
Fruit, mixed, frozen (*Big Valley*), ⅔ cup 60
Fruit bar, frozen (see also "Ice bar" and "Yogurt bar"),
    1 bar:
all flavors (*Minute Maid* Fruit Juice), 2.25-oz. bar 60
all flavors (*Minute Maid* Juice), 1.75-oz. bar 50
all flavors (*Popsicle* All Natural) 50
banana cream (*Frozfruit*) 150
cantaloupe (*Frozfruit*) 60
cherry (*Frozfruit*) 70
coconut cream (*Frozfruit*) 170
cranberry-apple or guava pineapple (*Frozfruit*) 80
kiwi-strawberry (*Frozfruit*) 90
lemon, iced tea (*Frozfruit*) 80
lemon or lime (*Frozfruit*) 90

Fruit bar, frozen *(cont.)*

orange (*Frozfruit*) 90
orange (*Minute Maid*), 3.75-oz. bar 90
piña colada, cream (*Frozfruit*) 170
pineapple (*Frozfruit*) 80
raspberry or strawberry (*Frozfruit*) 80
strawberry (*Minute Maid*), 3.75-oz. bar 120
strawberry cream (*Frozfruit*) 130
strawberry-banana cream (*Frozfruit*) 140
tropical (*Frozfruit*) 90
watermelon (*Frozfruit*) 50

Fruit cocktail, canned, ½ cup:

in extra light syrup (*Del Monte* Lite) 60
in juice (*Del Monte* Naturals) 60
in heavy syrup (*Del Monte*) 100
honey flavor (*Del Monte* Natural) 80

Fruit drink blends (see also "Soft drinks" and specific
   listings):

(*Capri Sun Mountain Cooler*), 6.75 fl. oz. 100
(*Capri Sun Pacific Cooler*), 6.75 fl. oz. 100
(*Capri Sun Surfer Cooler*), 6.75 fl. oz. 100
(*Hi-C Ecto Cooler*), 8 fl. oz. 120
(*Tropicana*), 8 fl. oz. 130
(*Veryfine* Avalanche), 8 fl. oz. 110
(*Veryfine* Tropical Breeze), 8 fl. oz. 120
all flavors (*Shasta Plus*), 12 fl. oz. 170
punch (*Capri Sun*), 6.75 fl. oz. 100
punch (*Capri Sun Maui/Safari*), 6.75 fl. oz. 100
punch (*Minute Maid/Minute Maid* Box), 8 fl. oz. 120
punch, tropical (*Minute Maid/Minute Maid* Box), 8 fl. oz. 120
punch, frozen* (*R. W. Knudsen* Tropical), 8 fl. oz. 120

Fruit juice blends (see also specific listings):

(*Season's Best* Medley), 8 fl. oz. 130
punch (*Apple & Eve Nothin' But Juice*), 8 fl. oz. 120
punch (*Tree Top*), 10 fl. oz. 150
tropical fruit, chilled or frozen* (*Dole*), 8 fl. oz. 140

Fruit pectin (*Sure·Jell*), ¼ tsp. 5
Fruit protector (*Ever-Fresh*), ¼ tsp. 5
Fruit snack, all varieties:

(*Fruit By the Foot*), 1 roll 80

(*Fruit Roll Ups*), 2 rolls 110
(*Gushers*), 1 pouch 90
(*Smart Snackers*), .5 oz. 50
(*Stretch Island*), 1 oz. 90
Fruit spreads (see also "Jam and preserves"), 1 tbsp.:
all varieties (*Simply Fruit*) 40
all varieties (*Smucker's* Homestyle) 45
and peanuts (*Smucker's* Super Spreaders) 40
Fudge topping, see "Chocolate topping"

G

FOOD AND MEASURE   **CALORIES**

Garbanzo beans, see "Chickpeas"
Garbanzo flour (*Arrowhead Mills*), ¼ cup 90
Garden salad, dill or marinated, (*S&W*), ½ cup 50
Garlic:
1 clove, approx. .1 oz. 4
crushed (*Frieda's*), 1 oz. 39
Garlic, minced, 1 tsp. 13
Garlic dip, 2 tbsp.:
Italian (*Marie's*) 180
roasted, and onion (*Marie's Fat Free*) 35
Garlic dressing (*Christopher Ranch*), 1 tbsp. 53
Garlic powder (*McCormick*), ¼ tsp. 3
Garlic salt (*Morton*), ½ tsp. 2
Garlic spread (*Lawry's* Ready-to-Spread), 1 tbsp. 100
Gefilte fish, drained:
(*Manischewitz* Gold Vegetable Medley), 1 ball, ⅙ carrot . 80
(*Manischewitz* Gold with Olives and Carrots), 1 ball,
  ¼ carrot 60
Gelatin dessert, all flavors:
(*Jell-O* Snacks), ½ cup 80
(*Jell-O* Sugar Free Snacks), 3.2 oz. 10
(*Kraft Handi-Snacks*), ½ cup 80
mix (*Jell-O* Sugar Free), ½ cup* 10
mix (*Jell-O*), ½ cup* 80
Gelatin drink mix, orange (*Knox*), 1 pkt. 40
Ginger, fresh:
trimmed root, 1 oz. 20
chopped (*Christopher Ranch*), 1 tsp. 15
Ginger, candied or crystallized (*Frieda's*), 1 oz. 96
Ginger, ground (*McCormick*), ¼ tsp. 2
Ginger, pickled (*Eden*), 1 tbsp. 15
Ginkgo nut, shelled:
raw, 1 oz. 52

canned, drained, 1 oz. 32
Gluten, see "Wheat flour"
Godfather's Pizza, 1 slice:
cheese, original crust:
   mini, 1/4 pie 131
   medium, 1/8 pie 231
   large, 1/10 pie 258
   jumbo, 1/10 pie 382
cheese, golden crust:
   medium, 1/8 pie 212
   large, 1/10 pie 242
combo, original crust:
   mini, 1/4 pie 176
   medium, 1/8 pie 306
   large, 1/10 pie 338
   jumbo, 1/10 pie 503
combo, golden crust:
   medium, 1/8 pie 271
   large, 1/10 pie 305
Goose, roasted, 4 oz.:
meat w/skin 346
meat only 270
Goose fat, 1 oz. 255
Goose liver, see "Liver" and "Pâté"
Gooseberry:
fresh, green (*Frieda's*), 1 oz. 11
canned, in light syrup (*Comstock*), 1/2 cup 70
Goulash seasoning mix (*Knorr Recipe*), 1 1/3 tbsp. 35
Granola, see "Cereal"
Granola and cereal bar, 1 bar:
(*Kudos M&M's*) 90
(*Kudos Snickers*) 100
(*Rice Krispies Treats*) 90
all varieties (*Kellogg's Low Fat*) 80
all varieties (*Nutri-Grain*) 140
all varieties (*Quaker Chewy Lowfat*) 110
chocolate chip (*Quaker Chewy*) 120
chocolate chip (*Rice Krispies*) 120
chocolate chunk (*Carnation Granola*) 140

Granola and cereal bar *(cont.)*
oats and honey (*Carnation* Granola) 130
oatmeal raisin (*Sweet Success*) 120
peanut butter–chocolate chip (*Quaker Chewy*) 120
Grape:
fresh (*Dole*), 1½ cups 85
fresh, American type (slipskin), 10 medium 15
fresh, European type (adherent skin), seedless, 10
medium 36
canned, seedless, in heavy syrup (*Comstock*), ½ cup . . . 100
canned, Thompson seedless (*S&W* Fancy Jubilee),
½ cup 130
Grape drink, 8 fl. oz.:
(*Hi-C*) 120
(*Lincoln*) 130
punch, chilled or frozen* (*Minute Maid*) 120
frozen* (*Bright & Early*) 140
frozen*, white cocktail (*Seneca*) 130
Grape juice:
(*Goya*), 8 fl. oz. 140
(*Season's Best*), 8 fl. oz. 160
purple or white (*Seneca*), 8 fl. oz. 160
frozen (*Seneca*), 2 oz. 160
Grape leaves, stuffed (*Perfecta* Dolmadakia), 4.35 oz. . . 220
Grapefruit:
fresh (*Dole*), ½ medium 50
fresh, pink or red, California or Arizona, ½ medium 46
fresh, pink or red, Florida, ½ medium 37
fresh, white, California, ½ medium 43
fresh, white, Florida, ½ medium 38
in jars, pink or white, in juice (*Sunfresh*), ½ cup 45
Grapefruit drink, 8 fl. oz.:
pink (*Ocean Spray*) 110
ruby red (*Ocean Spray*) 130
ruby red and tangerine (*Ocean Spray*) 130
Grapefruit juice:
(*Ocean Spray*), 8 fl. oz. 100
(*S&W*), 6 fl. oz. 80
ruby red (*Tropicana* Carton/Plastic), 8 fl. oz. 100
frozen* (*Minute Maid*), 8 fl. oz. 100

Gravy, see specific listings

Great northern beans:

boiled (*Goya*), ¼ cup 70

canned (*Goya*), ½ cup 80

canned (*Green Giant/Joan of Arc*), ½ cup 100

canned (*Sun-Vista*), ½ cup 70

Green bean and mushroom casserole, frozen

   (*Stouffer's*), 3.8 oz. 140

Green beans, ½ cup, except as noted:

fresh, raw (*Dole*), ¾ cup, 3 oz. 25

fresh, boiled, drained 22

canned (*Allens* Shells Out) 30

canned, all varieties, except Italian cut (*Del Monte*) 20

canned, whole (*Green Giant*) 25

canned, cut (*Allens/Sunshine/Alma/Crest Top*) 30

canned, French style (*Allens*) 25

canned, Italian cut (*Allens/Sunshine*) 35

canned, Italian cut (*Del Monte*) 30

canned, w/potatoes (*Allens/Sunshine*) 35

frozen, whole (*Birds Eye*), 3 oz. 20

frozen, cut or French cut (*Birds Eye*), ⅔ cup 25

frozen, Italian (*Birds Eye*), ⅔ cup 35

frozen, and almonds (*Green Giant Harvest Fresh*), ⅔ cup . 60

frozen, w/potatoes, onions, and peppers (*Green Giant*

   American Mixtures) ¾ cup 45

Green peas, see "Peas, green"

Greens, mixed, canned (*Allens/Sunshine*), ½ cup 30

Grenadine syrup (*Mr & Mrs T*), 2 tbsp. 80

Ground cherry, trimmed, ½ cup 37

Grouper, meat only, 4 oz.:

raw 104

baked, broiled, or microwaved 134

Guacamole dip (*Nalley*), 2 tbsp. 120

Guacamole seasoning (*Lawry's*), ½ tsp. 5

Guava, pulp, ½ cup 42

Guava drink (*Mauna La'I*), 8 fl. oz. 130

Guava nectar (*Goya*), 12 fl. oz. 240

Guava paste (*Goya*), ¾" slice 100

Guava sauce, cooked, ½ cup 43
Guinea hen, raw, 4 oz.:
meat w/skin 179
meat only 125
Gyro mix (*Casbah*), ¹⁄₁₀ pkg. 64

H

FOOD AND MEASURE	CALORIES

Häagen-Dazs Ice Cream Shop:
ice cream, ½ cup:

butter pecan	320
Brownies à la Mode (*Extraas*)	280
Cappuccino Commotion (*Extraas*)	310
Caramel Cone Explosion (*Extraas*)	310
chocolate	270
chocolate Swiss almond	300
chocolate chip or coffee chip	290
chocolate chocolate, Belgian	330
chocolate chocolate chip or chocolate chocolate mint	300
chocolate peanut butter, deep	370
coffee cookies and cream	270
Cookie Dough Dynamo (*Extraas*)	300
macadamia brittle or *Midnight Cookies and Cream*	300
macadamia nut	320
pralines and cream	290
rum raisin	270
strawberry	250
Strawberry Cheesecake Craze (*Extraas*)	280
vanilla	270
vanilla fudge	290
vanilla Swiss almond	310
ice cream bar, chocolate, uncoated, 1 bar	200
ice cream bar, coffee or vanilla, uncoated, 1 bar	190

sorbet, ½ cup:

banana strawberry or orchard peach	140
chocolate or strawberry	130
mango, raspberry, or *Zesty Lemon*	120
sorbet, soft serve, mango or raspberry, ½ cup	100

yogurt, soft serve, ½ cup:

chocolate, nonfat, or vanilla, nonfat	110
chocolate mousse, nonfat	80

Häagen-Dazs, **yogurt** *(cont.)*

coffee 140

vanilla mousse, nonfat 70

Haddock, meat only, 4 oz.:

raw 99

baked, broiled, or microwaved 127

smoked 132

Haddock entree, frozen:

battered (*Van de Kamp's*), 2 pieces 260

breaded (*Van de Kamp's*), 2 pieces 280

breaded (*Van de Kamp's* Light), 1 piece 220

Hake, see "Whiting"

Halibut, meat only, 4 oz.:

Atlantic and Pacific, raw 124

Atlantic and Pacific, baked, broiled, or microwaved 159

Greenland, raw 211

Greenland, baked, broiled, or microwaved 271

frozen (*Peter Pan*) 110

Halibut entree, frozen, battered (*Van de Kamp's*),

3 pieces 330

Ham, fresh, meat only, 4 oz., except as noted:

whole leg, roasted, lean w/fat 333

whole leg, roasted, lean w/fat, diced, 1 cup 411

whole leg, roasted, lean only 249

whole leg, roasted, lean only, diced, 1 cup 309

rump half, roasted, lean w/fat 311

rump half, roasted, lean only 251

shank half, roasted, lean w/fat 344

shank half, roasted, lean only 244

Ham, cured, meat only, 4 oz., except as noted:

whole leg, roasted, lean w/fat 276

whole leg, roasted, lean w/fat, diced, 1 cup 341

whole leg, roasted, lean only 178

whole leg, roasted, chopped or diced, 1 cup 219

boneless (11% fat), roasted 202

boneless (11% fat), roasted, diced, 1 cup 249

boneless, extra lean (5% fat), roasted 164

boneless, extra lean (5% fat), roasted, diced, 1 cup . . . 203

Ham, refrigerated or canned, 3 oz., except as noted:

(*Black Label* Shelf) 110

(*Black Label* Refrigerated) 100
(*Curemaster* Half) 80
(*Jones Dairy Farm* Country Club/Family/Dainty) 100
(*Jones Dairy Farm* Old Fashioned) 220
(*Swift Premium*) 100
baked (*Louis Rich* Dinner), 3.3-oz. slice 80
honey or maple (*Jones Dairy Farm Country Carved*) . . . 100
slice (*Oscar Mayer*) 80
spiral sliced (*Jones Dairy Farm*) 180
steak (*Jones Dairy Farm Lean Choice/Rock River*) 100
steak (*Oscar Mayer*), 2 oz. 60
"Ham," vegetarian, frozen (*Worthington Wham*),
  2 slices 80
Ham bologna (*Boar's Head*), 2 oz. 80
Ham glaze (*Marzetti*), 2 tbsp. 35
Ham lunch meat:
(*Hormel Light & Lean* 97), 1-oz. slice 25
(*Hormel Light & Lean* 97 Deli), 2 oz. 50
all varieties, except cinnamon apple (*Healthy Deli*), 2 oz. . 60
baked (*Oscar Mayer*), 3 slices, 2.2 oz. 70
baked (*Oscar Mayer* Fat Free), 3 slices, 1.7 oz. 35
boiled (*Oscar Mayer*), 3 slices, 2.2 oz. 60
boiled (*Oscar Mayer Deli-Thin*), 4 slices 50
chopped (*Oscar Mayer*), 1-oz. slice 50
cinnamon apple grove (*Healthy Deli*), 2 oz. 70
cooked (*Alpine Lace*), 2 oz. 60
cooked (*Hormel* Deli/Low Salt), 2 oz. 60
honey (*Louis Rich Carving Board* Thin), 6 slices 70
honey (*Louis Rich Carving Board* Traditional), 2 oz. 50
honey (*Oscar Mayer* Fat Free), 3 slices, 1.7 oz. 35
honey or smoked (*Louis Rich* Fat Free), 2 slices 35
maple (*Patrick Cudahy*), 1-oz. slice 35
smoked (*Hormel Light & Lean* 97 Deli), 2 oz. 50
smoked (*Oscar Mayer*), 3 slices, 2.2 oz. 60
smoked (*Oscar Mayer Deli-Thin*), 4 slices 50
Ham patty (*Hormel*), 2-oz. patty 180
Ham salad spread (*Libby's Spreadables*), ⅓ cup 110
Ham spread:
deviled (*Underwood*), ¼ cup 160
deviled, w/crackers (*Red Devil* Snackers), 1 pkg. 310

Ham spread *(cont.)*
honey (*Underwood*), ¼ cup 190
honey, w/crackers (*Red Devil* Snackers), 1 pkg. 340
Ham and asparagus entree, frozen, bake (*Stouffer's*),
   9.5 oz. 520
Ham and cheese loaf (*Oscar Mayer*), 1 oz. 70
Ham and cheese patty (*Hormel*), 2-oz. patty 190
Ham and cheese sandwich, frozen:
(*Deli Stuffs*), 4.5-oz. piece 350
(*Totino's* Big & Hearty), 4.8-oz. piece 310
croissant (*Sara Lee*), 1 piece 300
Hamburger, see "Beef sandwich"
"Hamburger," vegetarian:
(*NewMenu* VegiBurger), 3 oz. 110
frozen, Southwestern black bean, or red pepper and
   garlic (*Fantastic Nature's Burger*), 2.5 oz. 110
frozen, grilled (*Fantastic Nature's Burger*), 2.5 oz. 120
frozen, ground (*Green Giant Harvest Burger* For
   Recipes), ⅔ cup 90
refrigerated (*Yves Veggie Cuisine*), 1 patty 83
mix (*Fantastic Nature's Burger* Original/BBQ), 1 patty* . . 170
Hamburger entree mix, 1 cup*, except as noted:
beef pasta (*Hamburger Helper*) 250
beef Romanoff or beef teriyaki (*Hamburger Helper*) 290
beef stew (*Hamburger Helper Homestyle*) 250
beef taco or cheddar melt (*Hamburger Helper*) 310
cheddar and bacon (*Hamburger Helper*) 350
cheese, three (*Hamburger Helper*) 340
cheeseburger macaroni (*Hamburger Helper*) 360
chili macaroni or pizza pasta (*Hamburger Helper*) 290
fettuccine Alfredo (*Hamburger Helper*) 300
Italian, cheesy (*Hamburger Helper*) 330
Italian, zesty (*Hamburger Helper*) 320
Italian rigatoni (*Hamburger Helper Homestyle*) 180
lasagna (*Hamburger Helper*) 280
meat loaf (*Hamburger Helper*), ⅙ loaf* 280
Mexican, zesty (*Hamburger Helper*) 300
mushroom and wild rice (*Hamburger Helper*) 310
nacho cheese (*Hamburger Helper*) 320
Oriental rice (*Hamburger Helper*) 310

pizza (*Hamburger Helper Pizzabake*), ⅙ pan* 270
potato au gratin (*Hamburger Helper*) 290
potato Stroganoff (*Hamburger Helper*) 270
Salisbury (*Hamburger Helper Homestyle*) 270
shells, cheesy (*Hamburger Helper*) 340
spaghetti (*Hamburger Helper*) 300
stew (*Hamburger Helper*) 250
Stroganoff (*Hamburger Helper*) 350
Swedish meatball (*Hamburger Helper Homestyle*) 300
Hash, canned (*Mary Kitchen* Fiesta), 1 cup 210
Hazelnut butter (*Roaster Fresh*), 1 oz. 188
Head cheese (*Oscar Mayer*), 1-oz. slice 50
Heart, braised or simmered, 4 oz.:
beef 199
chicken, broiler-fryer, or lamb 210
turkey 201
veal 211
Herbs, mixed (*Lawry's* Pinch of Herbs), ¼ tsp. 0
Herring, fresh, meat only:
Atlantic, raw, 4 oz. 180
Atlantic, baked, broiled, or microwaved, 4 oz. 230
lake, see "Cisco"
Pacific, raw, 4 oz. 224
Pacific, baked, broiled, or microwaved, 4 oz. 284
Herring, canned, see "Sardine, canned"
Herring, kippered, Atlantic, 4 oz. 246
Herring, pickled:
Atlantic, 4 oz. 297
in jars, drained (*Vita* Homestyle), 2 oz. 130
in jars, in sour cream (*Vita*), ¼ cup, 2¼ oz. 120
in jars, roll mops (*Vita*), 2½ oz., approx. 1 piece 140
Hickory nut, dried, shelled, 1 oz. 187
Hoisin sauce (*House of Tsang*), 1 tsp. 15
Hollandaise grilling sauce (*Knorr* Microwave), 2 tbsp. . . . 45
Hollandaise sauce mix (*French's*), 2 tbsp. 10
Home-style gravy mix:
(*Durkee*), ¼ cup* 15
(*French's*), ¼ cup* 10
(*Pillsbury*), ¼ cup* 10

Hominy, canned:

golden or Mexican (*Allens/Uncle William*), ½ cup 120

golden or white (*Van Camp's*), ½ cup 80

white (*Allens/Uncle William*), ½ cup 100

Hominy grits, dry, see "Corn grits"

Honey (*Aunt Sue's/Grandma's/Sue Bee*), 1 tbsp. 60

Honey bun, see "Bun, sweet"

Honey butter (*Downey's*), .5 oz. 60

Honey Dijon marinade (*World Harbors*), 2 tbsp. 35

Honey hickory sauce (*World Harbors* Ember Wisp),
  2 tbsp. 45

Honey loaf (*Oscar Mayer*), 1-oz. slice 35

Honey mustard sauce, California style (*Rice Road*),
  1 tbsp. 20

Honeycomb, strained (*Frieda's*), 1 oz. 86

Honeydew melon:

(*Dole*), 1/10 melon, 4.8 oz. 50

pulp, cubed, ½ cup 30

Horseradish, fresh, boiled, drained, chopped, ½ cup 13

Horseradish, prepared:

(*Kraft*), 1 tsp. 0

red, w/beets (*Gold's*), 1 tsp. 0

red, w/beets (*Hebrew National*), ½ cup 25

Horseradish sauce, 2 tbsp.:

(*Reese*) 100

(*Sauceworks*) 20

Hot dog, see "Frankfurter"

Hot fudge sauce, see "Chocolate topping"

Hot sauce, see "Pepper sauce" and specific listings

Hubbard squash:

raw (*Frieda's*), 1 oz. 14

baked, cubed, ½ cup 51

Hummus, 2 tbsp.:

(*Cedar's*) 50

dip, mix* (*Fantastic Foods*) 60

Hush puppies, frozen (*Stilwell*), 3 pieces 140

Hush puppy mix (*Martha White*), ¼ cup 120

Hyacinth beans, ½ cup:

fresh, boiled, drained 22

dried, boiled 114

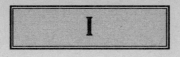

FOOD AND MEASURE   **CALORIES**

Ice, Italian:
cherry or lemon (*Marino's*), 4.7-oz. cup 100
Dutch cocoa (*Marino's*), 4.7-oz. cup 120
Ice bar (see also "Fruit bar, frozen"), 1 bar:
all flavors (*Popsicle*) 45
all flavors (*Popsicle* Sugar Free/Tropical Sugar Free) 15
cappuccino (*Frozefruit*) 140
cherry, lemon, and raspberry (*Good Humor* Hyper Stripe) . 80
cherry, lemon, and raspberry (*Popsicle* Firecracker) 40
lemon (*Great White*) 70
(*Popsicle Squeeze Ups*) 90
watermelon (*Good Humor*) 80
Ice cone (*Good Humor* Snow Cone), 1 cone . . . . , . 60
Ice cream, ½ cup:
almond caramel praline (*Breyers* All Natural) 170
almond, toasted (*Dreyer's Grand*) 150
banana split (*Edy's Grand*) 160
bananas Foster (*Healthy Choice*) 110
Black Forest or fudge brownie (*Healthy Choice*) 120
brownie, fudge (*Breyers Blends Sara Lee*) 190
brownie, fudge, à la mode (*Healthy Choice*) 120
brownie, fudge, double (*Edy's Grand*) 170
brownie, fudge, marble (*Breyers* Light/Lowfat) 120
butter almond (*Breyers* All Natural) 170
butter pecan (*Breyers* All Natural) 180
butter pecan (*Breyers* Light/Lowfat) 120
butter pecan crunch (*Healthy Choice*) 120
cappuccino (*Breyers Blends Maxwell House*) 170
cappuccino chocolate chunk (*Healthy Choice*) 120
cappuccino mocha fudge (*Healthy Choice*) 120
caramel praline crunch (*Breyers* Fat Free) 120
caramel praline crunch (*Edy's/Dreyer's* Fat Free) 120
cherry, black, swirl (*Edy's* Fat Free) 100

Ice cream *(cont.)*

cherry chocolate chip or espresso chip (*Edy's Grand*) . . 150
cherry chocolate chunk (*Edy's/Dreyer's Grand*) 150
cherry chocolate chunk (*Healthy Choice*) 110
cherry vanilla (*Breyers* All Natural) 150
Chiquita 'n chocolate (*Edy's/Dreyer's Grand* Light) 110
chocolate (*Breyers* All Natural) 160
chocolate (*Breyers* Fat Free) 90
chocolate (*Edy's/Dreyer's Grand*) 220
chocolate, triple (*Edy's/Dreyer's* No Sugar) 100
chocolate almond (*Breyers Blends Hershey's Almond*) . . 190
chocolate almond fudge (*Edy's/Dreyer's Grand* Light) . . . 120
chocolate brownie chunk (*Edy's/Dreyer's* Fat Free) 120
chocolate chip (*Edy's/Dreyer's Grand* Chips!) 160
chocolate chip, mint (*Breyers* Light/Lowfat) 110
chocolate chip, mint (*Edy's/Dreyer's Grand* Chips!) 170
chocolate chip, mint (*Healthy Choice*) 120
chocolate chip cookie dough (*Breyers* All Natural) 170
chocolate chip cookie dough (*Breyers* Light/Lowfat) . . . 110
chocolate chunk, triple (*Healthy Choice*) 110
chocolate fudge mousse (*Edy's Grand*) 160
chocolate fudge mousse (*Edy's/Dreyer's Grand* Light) . . 110
chocolate fudge mousse (*Healthy Choice*) 120
chocolate fudge sundae (*Edy's Grand*) 170
coffee (*Edy's/Dreyer's Grand*) 140
coffee fudge (*Edy's/Dreyer's* Fat Free) 110
cookie chunk (*Edy's/Dreyer's* Fat Free) 120
cookie creme de mint (*Healthy Choice*) 130
cookies 'n cream (*Breyers* All Natural) 170
cookies 'n cream (*Edy's/Dreyer's Grand* Light) 110
cookies 'n cream (*Healthy Choice*) 130
cookies 'n cream, mint (*Breyers* Fat Free) 100
cookie dough (*Edy's/Dreyer's Grand*) 170
cookie dough (*Edy's/Dreyer's Grand* Light) 130
espresso fudge chip (*Dreyer's Grand* Light) 120
French silk (*Edy's/Dreyer's Grand* Light) 120
fudge marble (*Edy's/Dreyer's* Fat Free) 110
fudge toffee parfait (*Breyers* Light/Lowfat) 120
Ice cream sandwich (*Edy's Grand*) 140
(*Milky Way*) 130

mocha fudge (*Edy's/Dreyer's* No Sugar) 90
mocha fudge, almond (*Dreyer's Grand*) 170
mocha fudge, almond (*Dreyer's Grand* Light) 120
mud pie (*Dreyer's Grand*) . . . . : . . 160
Neapolitan (*Dreyer's Grand*) 140
peach (*Breyers* All Natural) 130
peanut butter (*Breyers Blends Reese's Pieces*) 200
peanut butter caramel (*Breyers Blends NutRageous*) . . . 200
peanut butter cup (*Breyers Blends Reese's*) 210
peanut butter cup (*Edy's Grand* Light Cups!) 130
praline, almond (*Edy's/Dreyer's Grand*) 170
praline almond crunch (*Breyers* Light/Lowfat) 110
praline caramel or praline caramel cluster (*Healthy
   Choice*) 130
rocky road (*Breyers* Light/Lowfat) 120
rocky road (*Edy's/Dreyer's Grand*) 170
rocky road (*Edy's/Dreyer's Grand* Light) 110
rocky road (*Healthy Choice*) 140
rocky road deluxe (*Breyers* All Natural) 190
(*Snickers*) 220
strawberry (*Breyers* All Natural) 130
strawberry (*Breyers* Fat Free) 90
strawberry shortcake (*Healthy Choice*) 120
toffee bar crunch (*Breyers* All Natural) 170
vanilla (*Breyers* All Natural) 150
vanilla (*Breyers* Light/Lowfat) 130
vanilla (*Edy's/Dreyer's* Fat Free) 100
vanilla or vanilla and chocolate (*Edy's/Dreyer's Grand*) . . 150
vanilla, French (*Breyers* All Natural) 170
vanilla, French (*Breyers* Light/Lowfat) 90
vanilla bean (*Edy's/Dreyer's Grand*) 130
vanilla and black cherry (*Breyers Take Two* All Natural) . . 150
vanilla caramel (*Edy's/Dreyer's* Fat Free/No Sugar) 100
vanilla chocolate swirl (*Edy's/Dreyer's* Fat Free/No Sugar) . 90
vanilla-chocolate-strawberry combination (*Edy's Grand*) 140
vanilla fudge twirl (*Breyers* Fat Free) 110
vanilla and orange sherbet (*Breyers Take Two* All Natural) 140
vanilla and strawberry (*Breyers Take Two* Fat Free) 90
"Ice cream," nondairy, ½ cup, except as noted:
all flavors (*Tofutti* Soft Serve) 190

"Ice cream," nondairy *(cont.)*

all flavors (*Tofutti* Soft Serve Lite) 90
all fruit flavors (*Tofutti Fruitti*) 100
bar, chocolate or vanilla (*Rice Dream*), 1 piece 270
bar, strawberry (*Rice Dream*), 1 piece 250
better pecan (*Tofutti*) 220
cappuccino or carob (*Rice Dream*) 150
carob almond or mint carob chip (*Rice Dream*) 170
cherry vanilla (*Rice Dream*) 150
chocolate (*Tofutti*) 180
chocolate or cocoa marble fudge (*Rice Dream*) 150
chocolate chip or mint chocolate chip (*Rice Dream*) . . . 170
chocolate fudge or vanilla fudge (*Tofutti* Low Fat) 120
coffee marshmallow (*Tofutti* Low Fat) 100
cookies n' dream (*Rice Dream*) 170
Neapolitan or orange vanilla swirl (*Rice Dream*) 150
passion island fruit or peach mango (*Tofutti* Low Fat) . . 100
pie, cookie, all flavors (*Rice Dream*), 1 piece 320
pie, vanilla, chocolate covered (*Tofutti Cutie*), 1 piece . . . 250
strawberry (*Rice Dream*) 140
strawberry-banana (*Tofutti* Low Fat) 100
vanilla (*Rice Dream*) 150
vanilla or vanilla fudge (*Tofutti*) 190
vanilla almond bark (*Tofutti*) 210
vanilla Swiss almond (*Rice Dream*) 180
wildberry (*Tofutti*) 190

Ice cream bar, 1 bar, except as noted:

all flavors (*Fudgsicle* Pop Variety Pack), 1.75-oz. pop 60
almond (*Breyers*) 300
almond (*Good Humor*), 3.75-oz. bar 230
caramel crunch (*Klondike*) 300
chocolate (*Fudgsicle* Bar Fat Free), 1.75-oz. bar 60
chocolate (*Klondike*) 280
chocolate (*Weight Watchers Chocolate Treat*) 100
chocolate candy center (*Good Humor* Crunch) 280
chocolate cookie dough (*Ben & Jerry's*) 420
chocolate éclair (*Good Humor*), 3.75-oz. bar 220
coffee (*Klondike*) 290
cookies 'n cream (*Edy's/Dreyer's*) 250
(*Klondike*) 310

(*Klondike* Krispy) 300
(*Klondike* Krunch), 3.75-oz. bar 250
peanut butter (*Reese's NutRageous*) 240
strawberry shortcake (*Good Humor*), 3.75-oz. bar 210
toffee crunch, English (*Weight Watchers*) 110
vanilla (*Breyers*) 300
vanilla (*Good Humor* Premium), 3.75-oz. bar 220
vanilla (*Klondike* Original) 290
vanilla (*Klondike* Reduced Fat–No Sugar Added) 190
vanilla w/almonds (*Edy's/Dreyer's*) 270
vanilla, dark chocolate coated (*Klondike*) 290
vanilla, ice coated (*Creamsicle* Bar), 2.7-oz. bar 110
vanilla, ice coated (*Creamsicle* Pop No Sugar Added) 25
vanilla, milk chocolate coated (*Edy's/Dreyer's*) 250
vanilla and chocolate (*Good Humor* Number 1) 190
(*Weight Watchers Orange Vanilla Treat*) 40
Ice cream cone, plain, 1 piece:
cone, sugar (*Comet*) 50
cone, waffle (*Comet*) 70
Ice cream cone, filled, 1 cone:
butter pecan (*Breyers*) 300
chocolate dipped (*Good Humor* Premium Sundae),
    4.6 oz. 290
chocolate dipped (*Good Humor* Sundae), 4 oz. 230
chocolate dipped, w/peanuts (*Good Humor* American
    Glory) 230
cookies 'n cream (*Edy's/Dreyer's* Sundae) 250
vanilla fudge (*Edy's/Dreyer's* Sundae) 340
vanilla fudge ripple (*Good Humor* Choco Taco) 310
Ice cream cup, filled, 1 cup:
chocolate (*Sealtest*) 140
chocolate malt (*Milky Way*) 220
chocolate shake (*Milky Way* Lowfat) 220
(*Good Humor* Sundae Twist) 160
peanut butter (*Good Humor Reese's*), 3 oz. 220
strawberry (*Sealtest*) 130
sundae, chocolate chip cookie dough (*Weight Watchers*) . 180
vanilla (*Sealtest*) 140
vanilla (*Sealtest* Fat Free) 100
vanilla and chocolate (*Breyers*) 240

Ice cream loaf, all flavors (*Vienetta*), 2.4-oz. slice 190
Ice cream nuggets, chocolate coated:
(*Nestlé Crunch*), 8 pieces 310
dark (*Bon-Bons*), 5 pieces 190
milk (*Bon-Bons*), 5 pieces 200
Ice cream sandwich:
chocolate chip cookie (*Good Humor* Premium), 4 oz. . . . 280
(*Good Humor*), 3 oz. 160
Neapolitan (*Good Humor* Giant), 5 oz. 260
(*Weight Watchers*), 1 piece 150
Icing, see "Frosting"
Italian cut beans, see "Green beans"
Italian sausage, hot or sweet (*Perri*), 2.7-oz. link 230
Italian seasoning, 1 tsp. 3

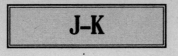

J–K

FOOD AND MEASURE   **CALORIES**

Jackfruit, trimmed, 1 oz. 27
Jalapeño, see "Pepper, jalapeño"
Jalapeño dip, 2 tbsp.:
(*Kraft*) 60
and cheddar (*Frito-Lay*) 50
cheese (*Kraft* Premium) 60
Jalapeño relish (*Old El Paso*), 1 tbsp. 5
Jam and preserves, 1 tbsp., except as noted:
all varieties (*Knott's Berry Farm*), 1 tsp. 18
all varieties, except mango (*Goya*) 45
all varieties, except grape and red plum (*Kraft*) 50
grape or red plum (*Kraft*) 60
mango (*Goya*) 46
orange marmalade (*Crosse & Blackwell*) 60
Java plum, seeded, ½ cup 41
Jelly (see also "Fruit spreads"), 1 tbsp., except as
   noted:
all fruit flavors (*Knott's Berry Farm*), 1 tsp. 18
all fruit flavors except apple and strawberry (*Kraft*) 50
apple or strawberry (*Kraft*) 60
grape (*Goya*) 45
guava (*Goya*) 50
pepper, mild (*Tabasco*) 60
pepper, spicy (*Tabasco*) 50
Jerk sauce (*World Harbors* Blue Mountain), 2 tbsp. 80
Jerusalem artichoke (*Frieda's Sunchoke*), 1 oz. 75
Jicama, see "Yam bean tuber"
Jujube, raw, seeded, 1 oz. 22
Jute, potherb, raw, ½ cup 5
Kale, ½ cup, except as noted:
fresh, raw, chopped (*Dole*) 17
canned (*Stubb's Harvest*) 25
frozen (*Seabrook*), 3 oz. 30

Kamut flour (*Arrowhead Mills*), ¼ cup 110
Kasha, see "Buckwheat groats"
Ketchup, 1 tbsp.:
(*Del Monte*) 15
(*Heinz*) 15
KFC, 1 serving:
chicken, *Original Recipe:*
   breast 400
   drumstick or whole wing 140
   thigh 250
chicken, *Extra Tasty Crispy:*
   breast 470
   drumstick 190
   thigh 370
   wing, whole 200
chicken, *Hot & Spicy:*
   breast 530
   drumstick 190
   thigh 370
   wing, whole 210
chicken, *Tender Roast:*
   breast, w/skin 251
   breast, w/out skin 169
   drumstick, w/skin 97
   drumstick, w/out skin 67
   thigh, w/skin 207
   thigh, w/out skin 106
   wing, w/skin 121
chicken potpie 770
Crispy Strips, 3 pieces 261
Hot Wings, 6 pieces 471
Kentucky Nuggets, 6 pieces 284
sandwiches, chicken:
   BBQ flavored 256
   Original Recipe 497
sides and specials:
   BBQ baked beans 190
   biscuit, 2-oz. piece 180
   coleslaw 180
   corn bread, 2-oz. piece 228

corn on the cob 190
garden rice 120
green beans 45
macaroni and cheese, 4 oz. 180
mashed potatoes w/gravy 120
Mean Greens 70
potato salad 230
potato wedges 280
red beans and rice 130
Kidney beans, ½ cup, except as noted:
dry, uncooked (*Arrowhead Mills*), ¼ cup 160
canned (*Seneca*) 110
canned, baked (*Friends*) 170
canned, dark or light (*Green Giant/Joan of Arc*) 110
canned, dark or light (*Van Camp's*) 90
canned, white (*Progresso* Cannellini), ½ cup 100
Kidneys, braised, 4 oz.:
beef 163
pork 171
veal 185
Kielbasa (see also "Polish sausage") (*Boar's Head*),
   2 oz. 120
Kishka (*Hebrew National*), 2 oz. 160
Kiwi:
fresh (*Dole*), 2 fruits, 5.3 oz. 90
fresh, fuzzless (*Frieda's*), 1 oz. 10
dried (*Sonoma*), 7–8 pieces, 1 oz. 90
Kiwi punch (*After the Fall* Bear), 8 fl. oz. 100
Knockwurst, beef (*Hebrew National*), 3-oz. link 260
Kohlrabi:
raw, sliced, ½ cup 19
boiled, drained, sliced, ½ cup 24
Kumquat, 1 medium, .7 oz. 12

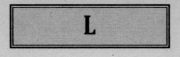

L

FOOD AND MEASURE   **CALORIES**

Lamb, choice, meat only, 4 oz., except as noted:
cubed, leg and shoulder, braised or stewed 253
cubed, leg and shoulder, broiled 211
foreshank, braised, lean w/fat 276
foreshank, braised, lean only 212
ground, raw 320
ground, broiled 321
leg, whole, roasted, lean w/fat 293
leg, whole, roasted, lean w/fat, 1 slice, 3″ diam. × ¼″ . . 73
leg, whole, roasted, lean only 217
leg, shank, roasted, lean w/fat 255
leg, shank, roasted, lean w/fat, 1 slice, 3″ diam. × ¼″ . . 64
leg, shank, roasted, lean only 204
leg, shank, roasted, lean only, 3″ slice 51
leg, sirloin, roasted, lean w/fat 331
leg, sirloin, roasted, lean w/fat, 1 slice, 3″ diam. × ¼″ . . 83
leg, sirloin, roasted, lean only 231
leg, sirloin, roasted, lean only, 3″ slice 58
loin chop, broiled, lean w/fat, 2.25 oz. (4.2 oz. raw
    w/bone) 201
loin chop, broiled, lean w/fat 358
loin chop, broiled, lean only, 1.6 oz. (4.2 oz. raw w/bone
    and fat) 100
loin chop, broiled, lean only 245
loin, roasted, lean w/fat 350
loin, roasted, lean only 229
rib, roasted, lean w/fat 407
rib, roasted, lean only 263
shoulder, whole, braised, lean w/fat 390
shoulder, whole, braised, lean only 321
shoulder, whole, roasted, lean w/fat 313
shoulder, whole, roasted, lean only 231

Lamb, New Zealand, frozen, meat only, 4 oz.:
leg, whole, roasted, lean w/fat 279
leg, whole, roasted, lean only 205
rib, roasted, lean w/fat 386
rib, roasted, lean only 222
Lamb entree, frozen (*Curry Classics*), 10 oz. 480
Lamb's-quarters, boiled, drained, chopped, ½ cup 29
Lard (*Goya*), 1 tbsp. 130
Lasagna entree, canned:
(*Libby's Diner*), 7¾ oz. 200
(*Nalley*), 7½ oz. 200
cheese, three, w/beef (*Nalley*), 7½ oz. 180
Lasagna entree, frozen, 1 pkg., except as noted:
(*Celentano* Great Choice), 10 oz. 260
Alfredo (*Weight Watchers*), 9 oz. 300
Alfredo, w/broccoli (*The Budget Gourmet* Special
    Selections), 9 oz. 380
bake (*Stouffer's*), 10¼ oz. 370
cheese, casserole (*Lean Cuisine Lunch Classics*),
    10 oz. 280
cheese, extra (*Marie Callender's*), 1 cup 330
cheese, five (*Stouffer's*), 10¾ oz. 360
cheese, three (*The Budget Gourmet*), 10.5 oz. 390
chicken (*Lean Cuisine*), 10 oz. 290
in meat sauce (*Freezer Queen* Deluxe Family), 1 cup,
    8.3 oz. 270
in meat sauce (*Freezer Queen* Homestyle), 10.5 oz. . . . 320
w/meat sauce (*Banquet* Bake at Home), 1 cup, 8 oz. . . . 240
w/meat sauce (*The Budget Gourmet* Light), 9.4 oz. 250
w/meat sauce (*Marie Callender's*), 1 cup, 8.9 oz. 350
w/meat sauce (*Smart Ones*), 9 oz. 240
w/meat sauce (*Stouffer's*), 10½ oz. 370
w/meat sauce, Bolognese (*The Budget Gourmet* Special
    Selections), 9 oz. 340
w/meat sauce, Bolognese (*Weight Watchers*), 9 oz. 300
mozzarella (*The Budget Gourmet* Special Selections),
    9 oz. 380
primavera (*Celentano* Selects), 10 oz. 210
sausage, Italian (*The Budget Gourmet*), 10.5 oz. 450
vegetable (*Amy's* Family), 7 oz. 200

Lasagna entree, frozen *(cont.)*
vegetable (*Stouffer's*), 10½ oz. 440
zucchini (*Healthy Choice*), 13.5 oz. 330
Lasagna entree mix:
(*Master-A-Meal*), ⅕ pkg. 150
tomato and vegetable (*Pasta Roni*), approx. 1 cup* 230
Leek:
fresh, raw, trimmed, chopped, ½ cup 32
fresh, boiled, drained, chopped, ½ cup 16
freeze-dried, 1 tbsp. 1
Lemon, fresh (*Dole*), 1 lemon 18
Lemon juice:
fresh, 1 tbsp. 4
bottled (*ReaLemon*), 1 tsp. 0
Lemon peel, candied, diced (*Paradise/White Swan*),
  2 tbsp. 80
Lemon sauce, pepper garlic (*World Harbors*), 2 tbsp. . . 35
Lemonade, 8 fl. oz.:
(*R. W. Knudsen*) 120
(*Tropicana*) 120
pink or frozen* (*Minute Maid*) 110
Lemonade fruit blends, 8 fl. oz.:
all fruit flavors (*Minute Maid*) 120
cranberry (*Heinke's*) 120
ginger (*R. W. Knudsen* Echinecea) 100
frozen*, all flavors except tropical (*Minute Maid*) 110
frozen*, tropical (*Minute Maid*) 120
Lemonade mix*, 8 fl. oz.:
(*Crystal Light*) 5
(*Kool-Aid* Presweetened) 70
Lentil, dry, green or red (*Arrowhead Mills*), ¼ cup 150
Lentil, canned (*Eden* Organic), ½ cup 90
Lentil, sprouted, raw, ½ cup 40
Lentil dishes, canned (*Patak's* Moong Dhal), ½ cup . . . 160
Lentil dishes, mix:
burgoo, spicy (*Buckeye Beans*), 2½ tbsp. 110
burgoo, spicy (*Buckeye Beans*), 1 cup* 200
cassoulet, sausage (*Buckeye Beans*), 2½ tbsp. 110
cassoulet, sausage (*Buckeye Beans*), 1 cup* 170
honey baked (*Buckeye Beans*), 4 tbsp. 180

honey baked (*Buckeye Beans*), 1 cup* 250
pilaf (*Near East*), 1 cup* 210
Lettuce (see also "Salad blend mix"):
Bibb or Boston, 2 inner leaves 2
cos or romaine, shredded, ½ cup 4
iceberg (*Dole*), ⅙ medium head, 3.2 oz. 15
iceberg, precut (*Dole*), 3 oz. 15
leaf, shredded (*Dole*), 1½ cups, 3 oz. 15
loose leaf, shredded, ½ cup 5
Lima beans, ½ cup, except as noted:
fresh, boiled, drained 104
fresh, mature, baby, boiled 115
fresh, mature, large, boiled 108
canned (*Green Giant/Joan of Arc* Butterbeans) 90
canned (*Stubb's Harvest* Butter Beans) 120
canned (*Van Camp's* Butterbeans) 110
canned, green (*Goya*) 90
canned, w/ham and sauce (*Nalley*), 1 cup 240
frozen, baby (*Birds Eye*) 130
frozen, Fordhook (*Birds Eye*) 100
Lime (*Dole*), 1 medium, 2.4 oz. 20
Lime juice:
fresh, 1 tbsp. 4
bottled or chilled (*ReaLime*), 1 tsp. 0
sweetened (*Rose's*), 1 tsp. 10
Lime drink, 8 fl. oz.:
(*R. W. Knudsen* Cactus Cooler) 120
frozen* (*Minute Maid* Limeade) 100
Ling, meat only, 4 oz.:
raw 99
baked, broiled, or microwaved 126
Lingcod, meat only, 4 oz.:
raw 96
baked, broiled, or microwaved 124
Linguine, plain:
dry, see "Pasta"
refrigerated, plain or herb (*Di Giorno*), 2.5 oz. 190
Linguine entree, frozen, 1 pkg.:
w/shrimp, clams (*The Budget Gourmet* Light),
    9.5 oz. 280

Linguine entree, frozen *(cont.)*
w/shrimp, clams, marinara (*The Budget Gourmet*),
9 oz. 270
w/tomato sauce and sausage (*The Budget Gourmet*
Special Selections), 10¼ oz. 380
Linguine entree mix, approx. 1 cup*:
chicken and broccoli (*Pasta Roni*) 370
chicken Parmesan, creamy (*Pasta Roni*) 410
Liquor[1], 1 fl. oz.:
80 proof 65
90 proof 74
100 proof 83
Liver:
beef, panfried, 4 oz. 246
chicken, raw (*Tyson*), 4 oz. 140
chicken, simmered, 4 oz. 178
duck, raw, 1 oz. 39
goose, raw, 1 oz. 38
lamb, panfried, 4 oz. 270
pork, braised, 4 oz. 187
turkey, simmered, 4 oz. 192
veal (calves), braised, 4 oz. 187
Liver cheese (*Oscar Mayer*), 1.3-oz. slice 120
Liver pâté, see "Pâté"
Liverwurst (see also "Braunschweiger"), 2 oz. or
¼ cup:
(*Boar's Head* Strassburger/Smoked) 170
pâté (*Boar's Head*) 150
spread (*Underwood*) 190
Lobster, northern, meat only:
boiled or steamed, 4 oz. 111
boiled or steamed, 1 cup, 5.1 oz. 142
frozen, chunks (*Tyson* Delight), 3 oz. 80
"Lobster," imitation, frozen or refrigerated:
chunks (*Louis Kemp Lobster Delights*), ½ cup, 3 oz. 80
tail style (*Captain Jac Lobster Tasties*), 4-oz. tail 120
Lobster sauce, rock (*Progresso*), ½ cup 100

---

[1] *Includes all pure distilled liquors (bourbon, brandy, gin, rum, Scotch, tequila, vodka, whiskey, etc.).*

Loganberry:
fresh, 1 cup 89
frozen, ½ cup 40
Longan, shelled:
fresh, seeded, 1 oz. 17
dried, 1 oz. 81
Loquat, 1 medium, .6 oz. 5
Lotus root:
raw, trimmed, 1 oz. 16
boiled, drained, 4 oz. 75
Lox, see "Salmon, smoked"
Lunch combinations (*Lunchables*), 1 pkg.:
bologna/American 470
bologna/wild cherry 530
chicken/turkey deluxe 390
ham/cheddar 360
ham/Swiss 340
ham/fruit punch 440
ham/fruit punch, low fat 350
ham/*Surfer Cooler* 390
pizza, mozzarella/fruit punch 450
pizza/pepperoni, mozzarella 330
pizza/pepperoni, orange 450
pizza, two cheese 300
salami/American 430
turkey/cheddar 350
turkey/ham deluxe 370
turkey/Monterey Jack 350
turkey/*Pacific Cooler* 450
turkey/*Pacific Cooler,* low fat 360
turkey/*Surfer Cooler* 430
Lunch meat (see also specific listings):
spiced loaf (*Oscar Mayer*), 1-oz. slice 70
canned (*Spam/Spam* Less Salt), 2 oz. 170
canned (*Spam* Lite), 2 oz. 110
canned, spread (*Spam*), 2 oz. 100
Lupin, boiled, ½ cup 98
Lychee, raw, shelled, peeled (*Frieda's*), 1 oz. 18

M

Macadamia nut:
dried, ½ cup 470
oil-roasted, 1 oz. 204
Macaroni (see also "Pasta"):
uncooked, elbow, regular or whole wheat (*Eden*),
  2 oz. 210
cooked, elbow, 1 cup 197
cooked, small shells, 1 cup 162
cooked, spirals, 1 cup 189
Macaroni entree, canned (see also "Chili"):
and beef (*Nalley*), 1 cup 220
and cheese (*Franco-American*), 1 cup 200
and cheese (*Nalley*), 7½ oz. 250
Macaroni entree, frozen:
and beef (*Banquet* Bake at Home), 1 cup, 8 oz. 230
and beef (*Freezer Queen* Homestyle), 9 oz. 220
and beef (*Marie Callender's*), 1 cup, 7 oz. 310
and cheese (*Banquet*), 10.5 oz. 350
and cheese (*The Budget Gourmet* Value Classics),
  9 oz. 380
and cheese (*Freezer Queen* Family Side Dish), 1 cup,
  8.6 oz. 240
and cheese (*Healthy Choice*), 9 oz. 290
and cheese (*Lean Cuisine*), 10 oz. 290
and cheese (*Marie Callender's*), 1 cup, 6.5 oz. 420
and cheese (*Smart Ones*), 9 oz. 220
and cheese (*Weight Watchers*), 9 oz. 300
and cheese, broccoli (*Lean Cuisine Lunch Classics*),
  9¾ oz. 240
and cheese, broccoli (*Stouffer's*), 10.5 oz. 360
and cheese, cheddar and Romano (*The Budget Gourmet*
  Special Selections), 9 oz. 310

Macaroni entree mix, dry, except as noted:
and cheese (*Land O Lakes* Original), approx. 1 cup* . . . 400
and cheese, all varieties (*Kraft* Dinner), 2½ oz. 260
and cheese, Alfredo (*Annie's*), ½ cup 200
cheddar or Parmesan (*Fantastic*), ⅜ cup 200
shells (*Land O Lakes*), approx. 1 cup* 330
Mackerel, meat only, 4 oz.:
Atlantic, raw 232
Atlantic, baked, broiled, or microwaved 297
king, raw 119
king, baked, broiled, or microwaved 152
Pacific and jack, raw 179
Pacific and jack, baked, broiled, or microwaved 228
Spanish, raw 158
Spanish, baked, broiled, or microwaved 179
Mackerel, canned, boneless, drained, jack, 4 oz. 177
Mahimahi, see "Dolphinfish"
Mai tai drink mixer, bottled (*Mr & Mrs T*),
 4.5 fl. oz. 140
Malt beverage (*Goya*), 12 fl. oz. 280
Malted milk powder, natural or chocolate (*Nestlé*),
 3 tbsp. 90
Mammy apple, frozen, chunks (*Goya*), ⅓ pkg. 140
Mandarin orange, see "Tangerine, canned"
Mango:
fresh, peeled, sliced (*Dole*), ½ cup 54
dried (*Sonoma*), 2 oz. 180
in jars, in light syrup (*Sunfresh*), ½ cup 100
Mango drink, 8 fl. oz.:
(*Tree Top* More Mango) 120
tangerine (*Veryfine*) 110
Mango nectar (*Goya*), 12 fl. oz. 230
Manicotti entree, frozen:
cheese (*Celentano*), 10 oz. 450
cheese (*Stouffer's*), 9 oz. 380
cheese, three (*Healthy Choice*), 11 oz. 260
cheese, w/meat sauce (*The Budget Gourmet*), 10 oz. . . . 420
Florentine (*Celentano*), 10 oz. 220
Maple syrup (*Cary's/Maple Orchard's/MacDonald's* Pure),
 ¼ cup 210

Margarine, 1 tbsp.:
(*I Can't Believe It's Not Butter* Salted/Sweet) 90
(*I Can't Believe It's Not Butter* Light) 50
(*Land O Lakes Country Morning* Salted/Sweet) 100
(*Land O Lakes Country Morning* Light) 50
(*Nucoa*) 100
(*Weight Watchers* Light/Light Sodium Free) 45
soft (*Chiffon* Tub) 100
spread (*Kraft Touch of Butter* Stick) 90
spread (*Kraft Touch of Butter* Tub) 60
spread (*Shedd's Spread*) 70
spread, w/sweet cream (*Land O Lakes*) 90
squeeze (*Kraft Touch of Butter*) 80
whipped (*Chiffon* Tub) 70
Margarita mixer:
bottled (*Holland House/Mr & Mrs T*), 4 fl. oz. 130
frozen* (*Bacardi*), 8 fl. oz. 90
mix (*Bar-Tenders*), 2 pkts., .9 oz. 90
Marinade (see also specific listings), 1 tbsp.:
(*Stubb's Legendary Moppin' Sauce*) 30
hickory grill or teriyaki (*Adolph's Marinade in Minutes*) . . 20
lemon garlic (*Adolph's Marinade in Minutes*) 30
mesquite (*Adolph's Marinade in Minutes*) 45
Marshmallow topping (*Smucker's*), 2 tbsp. 120
Mayonnaise, 1 tbsp.:
(*Best Foods/Hellmann's* Real) 100
(*Best Foods/Hellmann's* Low Fat) 25
(*Kraft* Real) 100
(*Nalley* Real) 100
(*Nalley* Light) 50
(*Smart Beat Super Light* Reduced Fat) 35
dressing (*Kraft Free*) 10
dressing (*Kraft Light*) 50
dressing (*Miracle Whip* Salad) 70
dressing (*Smart Beat* Nonfat) 10
tofu (*Nayonaise*) 35
McDonald's, 1 serving:
breakfast biscuits:
   plain 260
   bacon, egg, and cheese 440

sausage 430
sausage and egg 510
breakfast dishes:
   burrito 320
   eggs, scrambled, 2 160
   hash browns 130
   hotcakes, plain 310
   hotcakes, w/syrup, margarine 580
   sausage 170
breakfast muffins:
   English 140
   Egg McMuffin 290
   Sausage McMuffin 360
   Sausage McMuffin w/egg 440
Danish and muffins:
   apple bran muffin 300
   apple Danish 360
   cheese Danish 410
   cinnamon roll 400
sandwiches:
   Arch Deluxe 550
   Arch Deluxe w/bacon 590
   Big Mac 560
   cheeseburger 320
   Crispy Chicken Deluxe 500
   Fish Filet Deluxe 560
   Grilled Chicken Deluxe 440
   hamburger 260
   Quarter Pounder 420
   Quarter Pounder w/cheese 530
Chicken McNuggets:
   4 pieces 190
   6 pieces 290
   9 pieces 430
McNuggets sauce, 1 pkt.:
   barbeque or honey 45
   honey mustard or sweet and sour 50
   hot mustard 60
   light mayonnaise 40
french fries, small 210

McDonald's (cont.)

french fries, large 450
french fries, *Super Size* 540
salad, garden 35
salad, grilled chicken salad deluxe 120
salad croutons, 1 pkg. 50
salad dressing, 1 pkg.:
   Caesar or reduced-calorie red French 160
   ranch 230
   vinaigrette, light 50
desserts and shakes:
   baked apple pie 260
   chocolate chip cookie 170
   ice cream cone, vanilla, reduced fat 150
   McDonaldland Cookies, 1 pkg. 180
   shake, chocolate, strawberry, or vanilla, small 360
   sundae, hot caramel 360
   sundae, hot fudge 340
   sundae, strawberry 290
   sundae nuts, ¼ oz. 40
Meat, canned (see also specific listings):
potted (*Goya*), ¼ cup 60
potted or deviled (*Libby's*), 3 oz. 160
Meat loaf dinner, frozen (*Freezer Queen* Meal), 9.5 oz.   260
Meat loaf entree, frozen:
tomato sauce and (*Freezer Queen* Family),
   ⅙ of 28-oz. pkg. 150
w/whipped potato (*Lean Cuisine*), 9⅜ oz. 240
w/whipped potato (*Stouffer's* Homestyle), 9⅞ oz. 330
"Meat" loaf mix, vegetarian (*Natural Touch*), ¼ cup . . . 100
Meat loaf seasoning mix (*Adolph's Meal Makers*),
   1 tbsp. 30
Meatball entree, frozen, 1 pkg.:
Italian style, w/vegetables, in wine (*The Budget Gourmet*
   Italian Originals), 10 oz. 280
and spaghetti, see "Spaghetti entree"
Swedish (*The Budget Gourmet*), 10 oz. 550
Swedish (*Healthy Choice*), 9.1 oz. 280
Swedish (*Stouffer's*), 10¼ oz. 480
Swedish (*Weight Watchers*), 9 oz. 300

Swedish, w/pasta (*Lean Cuisine*), 9⅛ oz. 280
Meatball stew, canned (*Dinty Moore* Cup), 7.5 oz. 250
Melon salad, in jars:
in extra light syrup (*Sunfresh* Lite), ½ cup 45
in light syrup (*Sunfresh*), ½ cup 90
Mexican beans (see also "Chili beans"), canned, ½ cup:
(*Old El Paso* Mexe Beans) 110
w/jalapeños (*Brown Beauty*) 120
Mexican dinner (see also specific listings), frozen:
(*Patio* Fiesta), 12 oz. 340
(*Patio* Ranchera), 13 oz. 410
Mexican style (*Banquet* Extra Helping), 22 oz. 820
Mexican entree (see also specific listings), frozen:
(*Banquet*), 11 oz. 400
combination (*Banquet*), 11 oz. 380
Mexican seasoning (*Goya* Sazon), ¼ tsp. 0
Milk, 8 fl. oz.:
buttermilk, cultured 99
whole, 3.3% fat 150
low-fat, 2% fat 121
low-fat, 2% fat, protein fortified 137
low-fat, 1% fat 102
low-fat, 1% fat, protein fortified 119
skim, nonfat 86
Milk, canned, 2 tbsp.:
condensed, sweetened (*Borden*) 130
condensed, sweetened, low-fat (*Borden*) 120
condensed, sweetened, skim (*Borden* Fat Free) 110
evaporated (*Pet*) 40
evaporated, skim (*Pet*) 20
Milk, chocolate, see "Chocolate milk"
Milk, dry, nonfat (*Carnation*), ⅓ cup 80
Milk, goat's (*Meyenberg*), 1 cup 140
"Milk," nondairy, 8 fl. oz.:
(*EdenBlend*) 120
(*EdenRice*) 110
Milk beverage, flavored (see also specific flavors):
Butterfinger (*Nestlé Quik*), 8 fl. oz. 200
shake, root beer (*Nestlé Killer*), 14 oz. 460

Milkfish, meat only, 4 oz.:

raw 168

baked, broiled, or microwaved 215

Millet, hulled (*Arrowhead Mills*), ¼ cup 150

Mincemeat, see "Pie filling"

Miso, 1 tbsp.:

(*Eden* Hacho/Shiro) 35

(*Eden* Organic Mugi/Genmai) 25

Molasses, all varieties (*Grandma's*), 1 tbsp. 50

Monkfish, meat only, 4 oz.:

raw 86

baked, broiled, or microwaved 110

Monosodium glutamate (*Tone's*), 1 tsp. 0

Mortadella, w/pistachios (*Boar's Head Cinghiale*),

2 oz. 170

Mousse, frozen:

chocolate (*Weight Watchers*), 2.75 oz. 190

triple chocolate caramel (*Weight Watchers*), 2.75 oz. . . . 200

Muffin, 1 piece, except as noted:

(*Arnold Bran'nola*) 130

banana nut, mini (*Hostess*), 3 pieces 160

blueberry (*Entenmann's*) 160

blueberry (*Entenmann's* Fat Free) 120

blueberry, mini (*Hostess*), 3 pieces 150

cinnamon apple or chocolate chip, mini (*Hostess*),

3 pieces 160

corn (*Sara Lee*) 260

English (*Pepperidge Farm*) 130

English (*Wonder*) 120

English, cinnamon raisin (*Pepperidge Farm*) 140

English, regular, oat bran, or sourdough (*Thomas'*) 120

English, 7 grain or sourdough (*Pepperidge Farm*) 130

Muffin, frozen or refrigerated, 1 piece:

banana nut (*Weight Watchers* Fat Free) 170

blueberry (*Weight Watchers* Fat Free) 160

bran, harvest honey (*Weight Watchers* Fat Free) 160

chocolate chocolate chip (*Weight Watchers*) 190

English, honey wheat (*Thomas'*) 110

raisin bran or corn (*Pepperidge Farm*) 150

Muffin mix, 1 piece*:

apple cinnamon (*Betty Crocker*) 140

banana nut (*Betty Crocker*) 150

blueberry (*Betty Crocker*) 140

blueberry (*Betty Crocker* Fat Free) 120

blueberry (*Duncan Hines*) 160

blueberry (*Duncan Hines* Bakery Style) 190

blueberry, wild (*Betty Crocker*) 170

bran, oat (*Martha White*) 200

chocolate chip (*Duncan Hines*) 190

chocolate chocolate chip (*Pillsbury*) 190

cinnamon streusel (*Betty Crocker*) 170

cinnamon swirl (*Duncan Hines*) 200

corn (*Gold Medal*) 160

honey pecan (*Martha White*) 180

lemon poppy seed (*Betty Crocker*) 190

oatmeal raisin (*Martha White*) 200

raspberry (*Martha White*) 180

raspberry swirl (*Duncan Hines*) 160

strawberry (*Pillsbury*) 180

Muffin sandwich, see "Egg breakfast sandwich"

Mulberries, 10 berries, .5 oz. 7

Mullet, striped, meat only, 4 oz.:

raw 133

baked, broiled, or microwaved 170

Mung beans:

dry (*Arrowhead Mills*), ¼ cup 160

sprouted, raw (*Jonathan's*), 1 cup 30

boiled, ½ cup 95

Mushroom:

fresh (*Dole*), 5 medium, 3 oz. 20

canned, all varieties (*Green Giant*), ½ cup 30

freeze-dried (*Tone's*), ⅓ cup 15

frozen, breaded (*Empire* Kosher), 7 pieces, 2.9 oz. 90

marinated (*Seneca*), 1 oz. 90

pickled (*Seneca*), 1 oz. 5

Mushroom, enoki, 1 large, 4⅛" long 2

Mushroom, oyster, fresh (*Frieda's*), 3 oz. 20

Mushroom, portobello:

fresh (*Frieda's*), 1 oz. 8

Mushroom, portobello *(cont.)*
dried (*Frieda's*), ½ oz. 13
Mushroom, shiitake:
fresh, raw (*Frieda's*), 3 oz. 20
cooked, 4 medium or ½ cup 40
canned (*Seneca*), ½ cup 25
Mushroom gravy (*Heinz Homestyle* Fat Free), ¼ cup 10
Mushroom gravy mix, ¼ cup*:
(*French's*) 10
brown (*Durkee*) 15
Mushroom salad, all varieties (*Seneca*), 1 tbsp. 5
Mussel, blue, meat only, 4 oz.:
raw 98
boiled or steamed 195
Mustard, prepared:
(*Grey Poupon* Deli/Dijon/Spicy), 1 tsp. 5
(*House of Tsang* Chinese), 1 pkt. 15
all varieties (*Nance's*), 1 tsp. 15
blend (*Best Foods/Hellmann's Dijonnaise*), 1 tsp. 5
Mustard greens:
fresh, raw, chopped, 1 oz. or ½ cup 7
canned (*Stubb's Harvest*), ½ cup 30
frozen, chopped (*Seabrook*), 3 oz. 30

N

FOOD AND MEASURE | CALORIES

Nacho dip, mild (*Guiltless Gourmet*), 2 tbsp. 25
Nacho dip mix, (*Knorr*), ½ tsp. 10
Navy beans, ½ cup:
canned (*Allens*) 110
canned, bacon or bacon/jalapeño (*Trappey's*) 110
Navy beans, sprouted, raw, ½ cup 35
Nectarine, fresh (*Dole*), 1 fruit, 5 oz. 70
New England sausage (*Oscar Mayer*), 1.6 oz. 60
Noodle, Chinese:
(*Nasoya*), 1 cup, 2¾ oz. 210
cellophane or long rice, dry, 2 oz. 199
chow mein (*Mee Tu*), ⅔ cup 120
crispy, wide (*La Choy*), ½ cup 150
egg, dried (*House of Tsang*), 2 oz. 200
rice (*La Choy*), ½ cup 120
Noodle, egg:
uncooked (*Creamette/Penn Dutch*), 2 oz. 210
uncooked (*Manischewitz*), 2 oz. 210
uncooked, all varieties (*Eden* Organic), 2 oz. 220
uncooked, yolk-free (*Borden*), 2 oz. 210
cooked, 1 cup 212
cooked, spinach, 1 cup 211
Noodle, Japanese, dry, except as noted:
soba (*Eden* Organic Traditional), ½ cup 200
soba, buckwheat (*Eden* 100%), 2 oz. 200
soba, buckwheat (*Eden* 40%), 2 oz. 190
soba, cooked, 1 cup 113
somen (*Eden* Organic Traditional), ½ cup 200
spinach (*Nasoya*), 1 cup, 2¾ oz. 210
udon (*Eden*), 2 oz. 190
udon, brown rice (*Eden* Organic Traditional), ½ cup . . . 200
Noodle dishes, mix, ½ pkg. dry, except as noted:
Alfredo (*Lipton* Noodles & Sauce) 250

Noodle dishes, mix *(cont.)*

Alfredo, carbonara, or broccoli (*Lipton* Noodles & Sauce)   260
beef (*Lipton* Noodles & Sauce)   220
butter (*Lipton* Noodles & Sauce)   260
butter and herb (*Lipton* Noodles & Sauce)   250
cheddar (*Kraft* Dinner), 2.5 oz.   270
cheddar (*Nissin* Noodles and Sauce), 2.5 oz.   330
cheddar, bacon (*Lipton* Noodles & Sauce)   230
cheese (*Lipton* Noodles & Sauce)   250
chicken/chicken flavor:
   (*Kraft* Dinner), 2.5 oz.   270
   (*Lipton* Noodles & Sauce)   230
   (*Nissin* Noodles and Sauce), 2.4 oz.   330
   broccoli or tetrazzini (*Lipton* Noodles &
     Sauce)   220
   creamy (*Lipton* Noodles & Sauce)   230
Oriental (*Knorr* Cup), 1 pkg.   210
Oriental (*Pasta Roni*), approx. 1 cup*   290
Parmesan (*Lipton* Noodles & Sauce)   250
Romanoff (*Lipton* Noodles & Sauce)   260
sour cream and chive (*Lipton* Noodles & Sauce)   260
Stroganoff (*Lipton* Noodles & Sauce)   210
tomato, Italian (*Nissin* Noodles & Sauce), 2.4 oz.   320
Noodle entree, canned, 1 cup, except as noted:
w/beef (*Hunt's* Homestyle)   150
w/beef (*La Choy* Bi-Pack)   150
w/chicken (*Dinty Moore*), 7½ oz.   200
w/chicken (*La Choy* Bi-Pack)   160
w/chicken (*Nalley* Dinner)   190
w/chicken, cacciatore or regular (*Hunt's* Homestyle) . . .   175
w/chicken and mushrooms (*Hunt's* Homestyle)   200
w/chicken and vegetables (*Nalley*)   160
w/chicken and vegetables (*Nalley*), 7½ oz.   140
w/franks (*Van Camp's Noodle Weenee*), 1 can   230
sweet and sour, with chicken (*La Choy* Entree)   260
w/vegetables (*La Choy* Entree)   130
w/vegetables and beef (*La Choy* Entree)   160
w/vegetables and chicken (*La Choy* Entree)   160
Noodle entree, frozen:
and beef (*Banquet* Family), 1 cup, 7 oz.   140

escalloped, and chicken (*Marie Callender's*), 1 cup,
6.5 oz. 270

escalloped, and turkey (*The Budget Gourmet* Special
Selections), 10¾ oz. 430

kung pao, and vegetables (*Weight Watchers* International
Selections), 10 oz. 280

Romanoff (*Stouffer's*), 12 oz. 490

Nuts, see specific listings

Nuts, mixed, 1 oz., except as noted:

dry-roasted (*Planters*) 170

honey-roasted (*Planters*) 140

oil-roasted (*Paradise/White Swan*), ¼ cup, 1.2 oz. 210

oil-roasted (*Planters*) 170

oil-roasted, no Brazils (*Planters* 3½ oz.) 170

oil-roasted, no peanuts (*Paradise/White Swan* Deluxe),
¼ cup, 1.2 oz. 220

sesame, oil-roasted (*Planters*) 150

tamari-roasted (*Eden*) 170

O

FOOD AND MEASURE	CALORIES

Oat (see also "Cereal"):

whole grain, 1 oz. 110

flakes, rolled (*Arrowhead Mills*), ⅓ cup 130

rolled or oatmeal, dry, 1 oz. 109

rolled or oatmeal, cooked, 1 cup 145

Oat bran, dry (*Arrowhead Mills*), ⅓ cup 150

Oat flour (*Arrowhead Mills*), ⅓ cup 120

Oat groats (*Arrowhead Mills*), ¼ cup 160

Ocean perch, Atlantic, meat only, 4 oz.:

raw 107

baked, broiled, or microwaved 137

Ocean perch entree, battered, frozen (*Van de Kamp's*),

   2 fillets 300

Octopus, meat only, boiled or steamed, 4 oz. 186

Octopus, canned, ¼ cup, except as noted:

in garlic sauce (*Goya*) 160

à la marinara (*Goya*) 180

in olive oil (*Goya*) 150

spiced, in red sauce (*Reese*), 2 oz. 120

Oheloberry, ½ cup 20

Oil, 1 tbsp., except as noted:

all varieties and blends (*Crisco*) 120

almond, canola, corn, cottonseed, hazelnut, olive, palm,

   peanut, poppy seed, safflower, sesame, soybean,

   sunflower, vegetable, or walnut 120

avocado or mustard 124

butter oil 112

coconut 117

cod liver or herring 123

Oriental cooking or sesame (*House of Tsang Mongolian*

   Fire/Saigon Sizzle), 1 tsp. 45

salmon or sardine 123

sesame, toasted or hot pepper (*Eden*) 130

wok (*House of Tsang*) 130
Oil substitute (*Baking Healthy*), 1 tbsp. 30
Okra, ¹/₂ cup, except as noted:
fresh, boiled, drained, sliced 25
canned, cut (*Stubb's Harvest*) 25
canned, cut, w/tomatoes and corn (*Allens/Trappey's*) 30
frozen, whole (*Seabrook*), 9 pods, 3 oz. 25
frozen, cut (*Stilwell*), ³/₄ cup 25
frozen, and tomatoes (*Stilwell*), ²/₃ cup 25
Old-fashioned loaf (*Oscar Mayer*), 1 oz. 70
Olive, pickled, ¹/₂ oz., except as noted
black, see "ripe," below
Calamata (*Zorba*), 5 pieces 90
green, Manzanilla, stuffed (*B&G*), 5 pieces 25
green, queen, stuffed (*Lindsay*), 2 pieces 15
green, queen, stuffed w/tuna (*Goya*), 4 pieces 25
green, queen/Spanish (*B&G*), 2 pieces 20
green, queen/Spanish (*Zorba*), 2 pieces 25
green, stuffed (*B&G*), 2 olives 15
green, salad (*B&G*), 2 tbsp. 25
ripe, pitted (*Lindsay*), 6 small, 5 medium, or 4 large 25
ripe, pitted (*Lindsay*), 1¹/₃ tbsp. chopped 25
ripe, w/pits (*Lindsay*), 5 medium or 4 large 25
ripe, oil-cured (*Krinos*) 70
ripe, Greek (*Krinos*) 35
Olive loaf (*Oscar Mayer*), 1-oz. slice 70
Olive salad, drained (*Progresso*), 2 tbsp. 25
Onion, mature:
fresh or stored, raw, chopped, 1 tbsp. 4
fresh or stored, Vidalia, raw, chopped (*Dole*), ¹/₂ cup 30
canned or in jars:
　　whole (*Green Giant*), ¹/₂ cup 35
　　cocktail (*Crosse & Blackwell*), 1 tbsp. 5
　　sweet, in sauce (*Boar's Head* Vidalia), 1 tbsp. 10
　　wild, marinated (*Krinos* Volvi), 1 oz. 15
frozen, whole, small (*Birds Eye*), 17 pieces 30
frozen, chopped (*Ore-Ida*), ³/₄ cup 25
frozen rings, see "Onion rings"
Onion, cocktail, see "Onion"
Onion, dried, minced, 1 tsp. 7

Onion, french fried, canned (*French's*), 2 tbsp. 45
Onion, green (scallion):
raw, trimmed, w/tops, chopped (*Dole*), ¼ cup, .9 oz. 10
freeze-dried (*McCormick*), ¼ tsp. 1
Onion, Welsh, trimmed, 1 oz. 10
Onion dip, 2 tbsp.:
creamy (*Kraft* Premium) 45
French (*Kraft* Premium) 50
French or green (*Kraft*) 60
French or toasted (*Breakstone's*) 50
Onion gravy, ¼ cup:
roasted, and garlic (*Pepperidge Farm*) 25
zesty (*Heinz* Home Style) 25
mix* (*French's*) 15
mix* (*Loma Linda Gravy Quik*) 20
Onion powder (*McCormick*), ¼ tsp. 3
Onion rings, frozen:
(*Ore-Ida* Classic/Gourmet), 4 rings 220
(*Ore-Ida* Onion Ringers), 6 rings 230
Onion salt:
(*Durkee* California), ½ tsp. 0
(*Tone's*), 1 tsp. 1
Onion sprouts (*Shaw's* Premium Salad), 2 oz. 11
Opossum, meat only, roasted, 4 oz. 251
Orange:
(*Dole*), 1 fruit 50
California navel, sections w/out membrane, ½ cup 38
California Valencia, sections w/out membrane, ½ cup . . 44
Florida, sections w/out membrane, ½ cup 42
Orange, in jars, in light syrup, sections (*Sunfresh*),
    ½ cup 70
Orange, mandarin, see "Tangerine"
Orange drink:
(*Capri Sun*), 6.75 fl. oz. 100
(*Hi-C*), 8 fl. oz. 120
Orange drink blends, 8 fl. oz.:
cranberry (*Tropicana Twister*) 130
cranberry (*Tropicana Twister* Light) 30
peach, raspberry, strawberry-banana, or strawberry
    guava (*Tropicana Twister*) 120

raspberry or strawberry-banana (*Tropicana Twister*
    Light) 35
Orange drink mix* (*Tang* Sugar Free), 8 fl. oz. 5
Orange juice:
(*Dole*), 10 fl. oz. 140
(*Tree Top*), 8 fl. oz. 120
(*Tropicana* Pure Premium), 8 fl. oz. 110
ruby red (*Tropicana* Pure Premium), 8 fl. oz. 120
frozen (*Seneca TreeSweet*), 2 oz. 110
Orange juice blends:
grapefruit, 6 fl. oz. 80
mango (*R. W. Knudsen*), 8 fl. oz. 120
punch (*Juicy Juice*), 8 fl. oz. 120
Orange juice float (*R. W. Knudsen*), 8 fl. oz. 140
Orange peel, candied, diced (*Paradise/White Swan*),
    2 tbsp. 90
Orange sauce, mandarin (*Ka-Me*), 2 tbsp. 80
Oregano, dried, 1 tsp. 3
Oriental sauce, see "Stir-fry sauce" and specific listings
Oyster, fresh, meat only:
Eastern, wild, raw, 6 medium, 3 oz. 57
Eastern, wild, baked, broiled, or microwaved, 4 oz. 82
Eastern, wild, steamed or poached, 4 oz. 155
Eastern, farmed, raw, 4 oz. 67
Eastern, farmed, baked, broiled, or microwaved, 4 oz. . . . 90
Pacific, raw, 4 oz. 93
Pacific, raw, boiled, or steamed, 1 medium 41
Pacific, raw, boiled, or steamed, 4 oz. 185
Oyster, smoked, canned (*Reese* Petite), 2 oz. 110
Oyster stew, see "Soup"

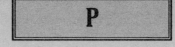

P

FOOD AND MEASURE   **CALORIES**

Palm, hearts of (*Goya*), ½ cup 25
Pancake, frozen, 3 pieces:
(*Aunt Jemima* Lowfat) 130
(*Aunt Jemima* Original) 200
blueberry (*Aunt Jemima*) 210
buttermilk (*Aunt Jemima*) 180
Pancake breakfast, frozen, 1 pkg.:
w/bacon (*Swanson Great Starts*) 400
w/sausage (*Swanson Great Starts*) 490
silver dollar, eggs and (*Swanson Great Starts*) 250
silver dollar, and sausage (*Swanson Great Starts*) 340
Pancake mix, ⅓ cup dry, except as noted:
(*Aunt Jemima* Original) 150
(*Aunt Jemima* Complete/Buttermilk Complete) 190
(*Betty Crocker* Complete/Buttermilk Complete) 200
(*Bisquick Shake 'N Pour*), ½ cup 210
(*Martha White Flapstax*), ½ cup 240
blueberry (*Bisquick Shake 'N Pour*), ½ cup 220
buckwheat (*Aunt Jemima*), ¼ cup 120
buttermilk (*Aunt Jemima* Complete Reduced Calorie) . . . 140
buttermilk (*Bisquick Shake 'N Pour*), ½ cup 200
corn, blue (*Arrowhead Mills*) 150
multigrain or whole grain (*Arrowhead Mills*), ¼ cup . . . 120
oat bran or wild rice (*Arrowhead Mills*) 140
Pancake syrup (see also "Maple syrup"), ¼ cup:
all varieties (*Aunt Jemima*) 210
all varieties (*Aunt Jemima* Lite) 100
butter or maple flavor (*S&W* Reduced Calorie) 60
Pancreas, braised, 4 oz.:
beef 307
lamb 265
pork 248
veal (calf) 290

Papaya:
fresh, peeled and cubed (*Dole*), ½ cup 27
dried (*Sonoma*), 2 pieces, 2 oz. 200
frozen, slices (*Goya*), ⅓ pkg. 50
in jars, slices, in light syrup (*Sunfresh*), ½ cup 70
Papaya, creamed (*R. W. Knudsen*), 2 fl. oz. 40
Papaya drink, 8 fl. oz., except as noted:
juice (*After the Fall* Pele's) 100
nectar (*Goya*), 12 fl. oz. 220
nectar (*R. W. Knudsen*) 130
punch (*Lincoln*) 130
Pappadum, snack crisps (*Tamarind Tree*), 30 pieces . . . 140
Paprika (*McCormick*), ¼ tsp. 2
Parfait, frozen, 1 piece:
double fudge brownie or praline toffee crunch (*Weight Watchers*) 190
strawberry (*Weight Watchers*) 180
Parsley, fresh, chopped (*Dole*), 1 tbsp. 10
Parsley root, 1 oz. 3
Parsnip, boiled, drained, sliced, ½ cup 63
Passion fruit:
fresh, purple (*Frieda's*), 3.5 oz. 90
frozen, chunks (*Goya*), ⅓ pkg. 70
Passion fruit juice, fresh, purple, 6 fl. oz. 95
Pasta, dry, uncooked (see also "Macaroni" and "Noodles"), 2 oz.:
all varieties (*Mueller's*) 210
all varieties, except angel-hair and garlic herb fettuccine (*San Giorgio*) 210
angel-hair or garlic herb fettuccine (*San Giorgio*) 200
fettuccine (*Prince*) 220
linguine, tomato-basil (*Prince*) 200
noodle-style, yolk free (*Mueller's*) 210
penne, tomato-pepper-basil (*Prince*) 210
spaghetti (*Prince* Square/Thin) 200
tricolor (*Mueller's*) 210
Pasta, dry, cooked, plain, 1 cup:
plain 197
corn 176
spinach 183

Pasta, dry, cooked *(cont.)*

whole wheat 174

Pasta, refrigerated (see also specific listings), plain,
2 oz.:

uncooked, w/egg 163

uncooked, spinach, w/egg 164

Pasta dishes, frozen (see also "Pasta entree, frozen"):

Alfredo (*Green Giant Pasta Accents*), 2 cups 210

cheddar, creamy (*Green Giant Pasta Accents*), 2⅓ cups 250

cheddar, white (*Green Giant Pasta Accents*), 1¾ cups . . 300

garden herb (*Green Giant Pasta Accents*), 2 cups 230

garlic (*Green Giant Pasta Accents*), 2 cups 260

Florentine (*Green Giant Pasta Accents*), 2 cups 310

primavera (*Green Giant Pasta Accents*), 2¼ cups 320

Pasta dishes, mix (see also specific listings):

broccoli, and mushroom (*Pasta Roni*), approx. 1 cup* . . 450

cheese, four, corkscrews (*Pasta Roni*), approx. 1 cup* . . 410

chicken, herb Parmesan (*Golden Saute*), ½ pkg. 230

chicken, stir-fry (*Golden Saute*), ½ pkg. 220

fagioli, w/white beans (*Fantastic* One Pot Meals),
½ cup 150

garlic, butter (*Golden Saute*), ½ pkg. 210

garlic, creamy, corkscrews (*Pasta Roni*), approx.
1 cup* 420

garlic, and herb (*Spice Islands* Quick Meal), 1 pkg. . . . 160

garlic, and olive oil (*Pasta Roni*), approx. 1 cup* 360

Mediterranean gemelli and red lentils (*Fantastic* One Pot
Meals), ⅜ cup 150

Parmesan (*Pasta Roni* Parmesano), approx. 1 cup* 390

primavera (*Spice Islands* Quick Meal), 1 pkg. 170

salad, Caesar (*Kraft*), 2.5 oz. 350

salad, garden primavera (*Kraft*), 2.5 oz. 280

salad, Italian, light (*Kraft*), 2.5 oz. 190

salad, Parmesan peppercorn (*Kraft*), 2.5 oz. 360

salad, ranch, classic, w/bacon (*Kraft*), 2.5 oz. 360

spinach and mushroom (*Spice Islands* Quick Meal),
1 pkg. 160

tomato, creamy, basil (*Spice Islands* Quick Meal), 1 pkg. 190

Pasta entree, frozen (see also specific listings):
bow ties, and creamy tomato sauce (*Lean Cuisine Lunch
  Classics*), 9.5 oz. 290
cheddar bake w/ (*Lean Cuisine*), 9 oz. 260
cheddar, w/beef and tomatoes (*Stouffer's*), 11 oz. 450
primavera, Alfredo (*Lean Cuisine Lunch Classics*),
  10 oz. 300
primavera, w/chicken (*Marie Callender's*), 1 cup,
  6.5 oz. 310
and sausage in cream sauce (*The Budget Gourmet* Italian
  Originals), 10.5 oz. 440
shells and cheese (*Stouffer*), ½ of 12-oz. pkg. 260
w/tomato basil sauce (*Weight Watchers* International
  Selections), 9.6 oz. 260
wide ribbon w/ricotta (*The Budget Gourmet* Special
  Selections), 10¼ oz. 430
wine and mushroom sauce, w/chicken (*The Budget
  Gourmet* Italian Originals), 10 oz. 290
Pasta flour, see "Semolina flour"
Pasta salad, see "Pasta dishes, mix"
Pasta sauce (see also specific listings), tomato, ½ cup:
(*Healthy Choice*) 50
(*Hunt's* Homestyle/Old Country) 55
(*Hunt's* Original) 65
(*Progresso*) 100
(*Ragú* Light No Sugar Added) 60
(*Ragú* Old World Traditional) 80
all varieties, except no sugar added (*Ragú* Light) 50
all varieties, except vegetable primavera (*Ragú*
  Gardenstyle) 120
w/basil (*Del Monte* D'Italia) 50
w/basil, summer tomato (*Five Brothers*) 60
w/basil (*Hunt's* Classic) 50
beef or beef and pork (*Porino's*) 120
cheese, four (*Del Monte* D'Italia) 60
cheese, wine and herbs (*Porino's*) 150
cheese and garlic, Italian (*Hunt's*) 65
fra diavolo (*Patsy's*) 120
garden style (*Del Monte*) 60
garden vegetable primavera (*Five Brothers*) 70

Pasta sauce *(cont.)*
garlic and herb (*Healthy Choice*) 50
garlic and herb (*Hunt's* Old Country) 65
garlic and onion (*Del Monte*) 60
garlic and onion (*Healthy Choice* Extra Chunky) 40
garlic and onion (*Hunt's* Chunky/Classic) 60
Italian herb (*Del Monte*) 60
marinara (*Del Monte* D'Italia Classic) 50
marinara (*Patsy's*) 120
marinara (*Progresso* Authentic) 90
marinara (*Ragú* Old World) 90
marinara, w/burgundy (*Five Brothers*) 80
meat/meat flavor:
   (*Del Monte*) 70
   (*Healthy Choice*) .50
   (*Hunt's* Homestyle/Old Country) 55
   (*Hunt's* Original) .65
   (*Prego*) 140
   (*Progresso*) 100
   (*Ragú* Old World) .90
mushroom:
   (*Del Monte*) 70
   (*Five Brothers*) 90
   (*Healthy Choice*) .50
   (*Healthy Choice* Extra Chunky) 40
   (*Hunt's* Homestyle/Old Country) 55
   (*Hunt's* Original) .65
   (*Progresso*) 80
   (*Ragú* Old World) .80
   (*Weight Watchers*) 60
   garlic (*Barilla*) 80
   garlic or sweet pepper (*Healthy Choice* Super Chunky)   45
olive, black, and mushrooms (*Porino's*) 100
w/Parmesan (*Hunt's* Classic) 50
pepper, red (*Del Monte* D'Italia) 50
sausage, Italian (*Hunt's*) 75
w/vegetables (*Hunt's* Chunky) 65
w/vegetables, Italian (*Healthy Choice* Extra Chunky) 40
w/vegetables, Italian (*Hunt's* Old Country) 65
w/vegetables, primavera (*Healthy Choice* Super Chunky) . .45

w/vegetables, primavera (*Ragú* Gardenstyle) 110
Pasta sauce, refrigerated, tomato base:
cheese, four (*Di Giorno*), ¼ cup 200
chunky tomato (*Contadina* Fat Free), ½ cup 45
garden vegetable (*Contadina* Fat Free), ½ cup 40
marinara (*Contadina*), ½ cup 80
marinara (*Di Giorno*), ½ cup 100
meat, traditional (*Di Giorno*), ½ cup 120
olive oil and garlic, w/cheese (*Di Giorno*), ¼ cup 370
red bell pepper (*Contadina*), ½ cup 180
tomato, basil (*Contadina* Fat Free), ½ cup 45
tomato, chunky, w/basil (*Di Giorno* Light), ½ cup 70
tomato, plum, and basil (*Contadina*), ½ cup 70
tomato, plum, and mushroom (*Di Giorno*), ½ cup 70
Pasta sauce mix (see also specific listings):
(*Knorr* Parma Rosa), 2 tbsp. 60
garlic and herb (*Knorr*), ⅓ pkg. 70
primavera (*Spice Islands* Pouch), ⅕ pkg. 30
spaghetti, American or mushroom (*Durkee*), ½ cup* 15
spaghetti, zesty (*Durkee*), 2 tsp. 20
Pastrami (see also "Turkey pastrami"), beef, 2 oz.:
(*Hebrew National*) 80
round (*Hebrew National*) 70
Pastry shell (*Stella D'Oro*), 1-oz. shell 140
Pastry shell, frozen (see also "Pie crust"):
dough (*Goya* Discos), 1 piece 120
patty (*Pepperidge Farm*), 1 shell 230
tart (*Pet-Ritz*), 3″ shell 140
Pâté, liver (see also "Liverwurst"), canned:
1 oz. 90
chicken liver, 1 oz. 57
goose liver, smoked, 1 oz. 131
(*Sells*), ¼ cup 160
"Pâté," vegetarian (*Bonavita* Swiss), 1 oz. 61
Pea pod, Chinese, see "Peas, edible-podded"
Peach:
fresh (*Dole*), 2 fruits 70
fresh, pulp, sliced, ½ cup 37
canned, ½ cup:
in juice, cling (*Del Monte* Naturals) 60

Peach, canned *(cont.)*
  in extra light syrup *(Del Monte Lite)* 60
  in heavy syrup *(Del Monte/Del Monte Melba)* 100
  raspberry flavor, cling, heavy syrup *(Del Monte)* 80
  spiced *(Del Monte Natural Harvest)* 80
  frozen *(Big Valley)*, ²/₃ cup 50
  sun-dried *(Del Monte)*, ¹/₃ cup, 1.4 oz. 90
Peach butter *(Smucker's)*, 1 tbsp. 45
Peach juice blend *(Dole Orchard)*, 8 fl. oz. 140
Peach nectar, 8 fl. oz.:
(Goya) 150
(R. W. Knudsen) 120
Peanut, shelled, 1 oz., except as noted:
unroasted 159
dry-roasted or honey-roasted *(Planters)* 160
honey-roasted *(Frito-Lay)*, ¹/₄ cup 270
honey-roasted *(Smart Snackers)*, .7 oz. 100
hot *(Frito-Lay)*, ¹/₄ cup 280
hot and spicy *(Planters Heat)* 160
oil-roasted *(Planters/Planters Munch 'N Go)* 170
oil-roasted, salted *(Frito-Lay)* 180
Spanish *(Planters)* 170
sweet *(Planters Sweet N Crunchy)* 140
Peanut butter, 2 tbsp., except as noted:
all varieties *(Peter Pan/Peter Pan Real)* 190
all varieties *(Peter Pan Whipped)* 150
creamy or chunky *(Jif/Simply Jif/Jif Reduced Fat)* 190
creamy, spread *(Peter Pan Smart Choice)* 180
crunchy, spread *(Peter Pan Smart Choice)* 195
and jelly *(Smucker's Goober)*, 3 tbsp. 230
Peanut butter caramel topping *(Smucker's)*, 2 tbsp. . . . 150
Peanut butter snack *(Mr. Peanut P. B. Crisps)*, 1 oz. . . . 140
Peanut sauce, Oriental *(Kylin Singapore Satay)*, ¹/₄ cup . . 60
Pear:
fresh *(Dole)*, 1 fruit 100
canned, ¹/₂ cup:
  in juice or extra light syrup *(Del Monte Naturals)* 60
  in juice or extra light syrup *(Del Monte Lite)* 60
  in heavy syrup *(Del Monte)* 100
  ginger flavor *(Del Monte Natural)* 90

dried (*Sonoma*), 3–4 pieces, 1.4 oz. 120
Pear juice (*R. W. Knudsen* Organic), 8 fl. oz. 120
Pear nectar (*Santa Cruz*), 8 fl. oz. 120
Peas, butter, frozen (*Stilwell*), ½ cup 110
Peas, cream, canned (*Allens/East Texas Fair*), ½ cup . . 100
Peas, crowder, ½ cup:
canned (*Allens/East Texas Fair/Homefolks*) 110
frozen (*Stilwell*) 120
Peas, edible-podded:
fresh, sugar snap (*Frieda's*), 1 oz. 15
frozen, sugar snap (*Birds Eye*), ½ cup 40
frozen, sugar snap, stir-fry (*Birds Eye*), ¾ cup 35
Peas, field, ½ cup:
canned, fresh shell (*Sunshine*) 120
canned, fresh shell, w/snaps (*Goya*) 110
frozen, w/snaps (*Stilwell*) 110
Peas, green:
fresh, raw, shelled, ½ cup 58
canned (*Del Monte/Del Monte* No Salt), ½ cup 60
canned, early June (*Sun-Vista*), ½ cup 80
canned, early or sweet (*Green Giant LeSueur*), ½ cup . . 60
canned, very young, small (*Del Monte*), ½ cup 60
dried (*Goya*), ¼ cup 100
frozen (*Birds Eye*), ½ cup 70
frozen, baby sweet (*Green Giant LeSueur*), ⅔ cup 60
frozen, early June (*Green Giant LeSueur*), ⅔ cup 60
frozen, tiny (*Birds Eye*), ½ cup 60
frozen, baby, butter sauce (*Green Giant LeSueur*),
   ¾ cup 100
Peas, green, combinations, ½ cup, except as noted:
canned, carrots (*Del Monte*) 60
canned, mushrooms, onions (*Green Giant LeSueur*) 60
canned, pearl onions (*Green Giant*) 60
frozen, carrots (*Stilwell*) 50
frozen, pearl onions (*Green Giant Harvest Fresh*) 50
frozen, potatoes, carrots (*Green Giant American*
   Mixtures), ⅔ cup 70
Peas, lady, canned (*Sunshine*), ½ cup 100
Peas, purple hull, canned (*Stubb's Harvest*), ½ cup . . . 120
Peas, split, see "Split peas"

Peas, sugar snap, see "Peas, edible-podded"
Peas, sweet, see "Peas, green"
Pecan, shelled:
halves or pieces (*Paradise/White Swan*), ¼ cup, 1 oz. . . . 200
honey-roasted (*Planters*), 1 oz. 180
Pecan topping (*Smucker's*), 2 tbsp. 190
Penne entree, canned, in meat sauce (*Franco-
   American*), 1 cup 240
Penne entree, frozen, 1 pkg.:
(*The Budget Gourmet* Special Selections), 9 oz. 290
Bolognese (*Lean Cuisine*), 9.5 oz. 270
spicy, and ricotta (*Weight Watchers* International
   Selections), 10.2 oz. 280
sun-dried tomato (*Weight Watchers*), 10 oz. 290
tomato sauce (*Healthy Choice*), 8 oz. 230
tomato basil sauce (*Lean Cuisine Lunch Classics*),
   10 oz. 290
Pepper, seasoning:
black, red, or cayenne, ground, 1 tsp. 6
chili, 1 tsp. 9
white (*McCormick*), ¼ tsp. 2
Pepper, frozen, stir-fry (*Birds Eye*), 3 oz. 25
Pepper, banana, hot or mild (*Vlasic*), 1 oz. 5
Pepper, bell, see "Pepper, sweet"
Pepper, cherry, hot (*B&G*), 1 oz. 10
Pepper, chili, raw, green and red:
1 medium, 1.6 oz. 18
chopped, ½ cup 30
Pepper, chili, in jars:
green, whole (*Nalley*), 1 oz. 10
green, chopped (*Old El Paso*), 2 tbsp. 5
green, diced (*Rosarita*), 2 tbsp. 5
Pepper, chili, relish, pickle (*Patak's*), 1 tbsp. 45
Pepper, jalapeño, whole or sliced (*Nalley*), 1 oz. 5
Pepper, serrano, canned (*Stubb's Legendary*), 1 oz. . . . 5
Pepper, stuffed, frozen (*Stouffer's*), 10 oz. 200
Pepper, sweet:
fresh (*Dole*), 1 medium 25
fresh, green (*Dole*), 1 medium, 5.3 oz. 30
fresh, yellow, raw, 1 large, 5″ × 3″ diam. 50

frozen, chopped, 1 oz. 6
Pepper, sweet, in jars:
(*B&G*), 1 oz. 10
fried, drained (*Progresso*), 2 tbsp. 60
red (*B&G*), 1 oz. 20
roasted (*Progresso*), 1 piece 10
sun-dried, marinated (*Antica Italia*), 1 oz. 170
Pepper dip, red (*Victoria*), 2 tbsp. 50
Pepper salad, drained (*Progresso*), 2 tbsp. 15
Pepper sauce, hot, all varieties (*Tabasco*), 1 tsp. 0
Pepper steak, see "Beef entree"
Pepper "steak" entree, vegetarian, frozen (*Hain*),
    10 oz. 310
Peppercorn sauce mix (*Knorr*), 2 tsp. 25
Pepperoncini:
(*Nalley*), 1 oz. 5
(*Progresso* Tuscan), 3 peppers 10
Pepperoni:
(*Boar's Head*), 1 oz. 140
(*Oscar Mayer*), 15 slices, 1.1 oz. 140
"Pepperoni," vegetarian (*Yves Veggie Cuisine*), 3½
    slices 78
Pepperoni bagel (*Hormel Quick Meal*), 1 piece 350
Perch (see also "Ocean perch"), meat only, 4 oz.:
raw 103
baked, broiled, or microwaved 133
Perch entree, frozen, battered (*Van de Kamp's*), 2 pieces 300
Persimmon:
native (*Dole*), 1 medium 32
dried (*Sonoma*), 6–8 pieces 140
Pesto sauce, ¼ cup:
in jars (*Sonoma*) 110
refrigerated (*Contadina* Reduced Fat) 230
refrigerated (*Di Giorno*) 320
Pesto sauce mix (*Spice Islands*), ¼ pkg. 15
Pheasant, raw, meat only, ½ breast, 6.4 oz. 243
Picante sauce (see also "Salsa"), 2 tbsp.:
all varieties (*Old El Paso* Thick 'n Chunky) 10
medium (*Nalley* Superba) 10
mild (*Nalley* Superba) 5

Pickle, cucumber, 1 oz.:
(*B&G Sandwich Toppers* New York Deli Style) 0
bread and butter (*B&G Sandwich Toppers*) 30
bread and butter, chips (*B&G*) 30
bread and butter, chips (*B&G* Unsalted) 25
cornichons (*Roland* Gherkins), 6 pieces, 1 oz. 5
dill, all varieties (*Nalley*) 5
kosher (*Hebrew National/Rosoff/Shorr's*) 4
sour, kosher (*Hebrew National/Shorr's* New Half Sours) . . 4
sour, kosher, garlic (*Hebrew National/Shorr's*) 3
sweet (*B&G* Mixed) 30
sweet, gherkins (*B&G*) 35
Pickle dip, dill (*Nalley*), 2 tbsp. 70
Pickle and pepper loaf (*Boar's Head*), 2 oz. 150
Pickle and pimiento loaf (*Oscar Mayer*), 1-oz. slice 80
Pickle relish, cucumber, 1 tbsp.:
dill, chunky (*Nalley*) 0
emerald, hamburger or India (*B&G*) 15
hot dog or tomato piccalilli (*B&G*) 20
India (*Heinz*) 20
sweet (*B&G*) 15
sweet (*B&G* Unsalted) 20
Pickled vegetables, see "Vegetables, mixed, pickled"
Pie, ⅙ pie, except as noted:
apple (*Entenmann's* Homestyle) 300
coconut custard or lemon (*Entenmann's*) 340
lemon meringue (*Entenmann's*), ⅕ pie 270
Pie, frozen:
apple (*Mrs. Smith's* 8"), ⅙ pie 270
apple (*Sara Lee* Homestyle), ⅛ pie 330
apple, Dutch (*Mrs. Smith's* Old Fashioned), ⅛ pie 310
banana cream (*Banquet*), ⅓ pie 350
Boston cream, see "Cake, frozen"
cherry, lattice (*Mrs. Smith's*), ⅕ pie 320
chocolate cream (*Mrs. Smith's*), ¼ pie 330
chocolate cream, French silk (*Mrs. Smith's*), ⅕ pie 410
chocolate mocha (*Weight Watchers*), 2.75-oz. pie 170
coconut cream (*Mrs. Smith's*), ¼ pie 340
coconut custard, (*Mrs. Smith's*), ⅕ pie 280
lemon cream (*Mrs. Smith's*), ¼ pie 300

lemon meringue (*Mrs. Smith's*), 1/5 pie 302
lemon meringue (*Sara Lee* Homestyle), 1/6 pie 350
mince (*Mrs. Smith's*), 1/6 pie 300
Mississippi mud (*Weight Watchers*), 2.45-oz. pie 160
peach (*Mrs. Smith's 8"*), 1/6 pie 260
pecan (*Mrs. Smith's 8"*), 1/6 pie 520
pumpkin, hearty (*Mrs. Smith's 8"*), 1/5 pie 250
pumpkin custard (*Mrs. Smith's 8"*), 1/5 pie 270
raspberry or strawberry-rhubarb (*Mrs. Smith's*),
   1/6 pie 280
strawberry (*Mrs. Smith's*), 1/5 pie 280
Pie, mix*, 1/6 pie:
chocolate silk (*Jell-O*) 310
coconut cream (*Jell-O*) 330
Pie, snack:
all flavors except cherry (*Hostess*), 4.4 oz. 440
cherry (*Hostess*), 4.4 oz. 450
Pie crust:
chocolate cookie (*Oreo*), 1/6 crust 140
cookie crumbs (*Nilla*), 2 tbsp. 70
graham, mini (*Ready Crust*), .8-oz. crust 120
graham crumbs (*Sunshine*), 2 tbsp. 80
shortbread (*Ready Crust 9"*), 1/8 crust 100
vanilla cookie (*Nilla*), 1/6 crust 140
Pie crust, frozen or refrigerated (see also "Pastry
   shell"):
(*Pillsbury*), 1/8 crust 120
deep dish (*Pet-Ritz*), 1/8 crust 90
vegetable shortening (*Pet-Ritz*), 1/8 crust 80
Pie crust mix:
(*Flako*), 1/4 cup dry 130
(*Pillsbury*), 1/8 of 9" crust 100
Pie filling, canned, 1/3 cup:
apple (*Comstock*) 100
apple (*Comstock* More Fruit) 80
apple, cinnamon 'n spice (*Comstock* More Fruit) 110
apple-cranberry (*Comstock*) 90
banana cream (*Comstock*) 130
blackberry (*Comstock*) 110
blueberry or apricot (*Comstock*) 100

Pie filling *(cont.)*
blueberry (*Comstock* More Fruit) 80
blueberry-cranberry (*Comstock*) 100
cherry (*Comstock/Comstock* More Fruit) 90
cherry (*Comstock* Lite/*Comstock* More Fruit Lite) 60
cherry, dark sweet (*Comstock*) 100
cherry-cranberry (*Comstock*) 90
chocolate cream (*Comstock*) 130
coconut cream (*Comstock*) 120
lemon (*Comstock*) 130
mince (*Comstock*) 170
mince, w/brandy and rum (*None Such*) 200
peach (*Comstock* More Fruit) 80
pineapple (*Comstock*) 110
pumpkin, mix (*Comstock*) 90
raisin (*Comstock*) 120
raspberry or strawberry (*Comstock*) 100
Pigeon peas:
dried (*Goya*), ¼ cup 140
canned, dried (*El Jib*), ½ cup 80
canned, green (*Tupi*), ½ cup 70
Pig's feet, pickled (*Hormel*), 2 oz. 80
Pignoli nuts, see "Pine nuts"
Pike, meat only, 4 oz.:
northern, raw 100
northern, baked, broiled, or microwaved 128
walleye, raw 105
walleye, baked, broiled, or microwaved 135
Pili nuts, dried, shelled, 1 oz. 204
Pimiento, drained (*Goya*), ¼ pepper 0
Piña colada mixer:
bottled (*Holland House/Mr & Mrs T*), 4.5 fl. oz. 180
frozen* (*Bacardi*), 8 fl. oz. 170
Pine nuts, dried, 1 oz.:
pignolia (*Progresso*) 170
pinyon 161
Pineapple, ½ cup, except as noted:
fresh, baby, trimmed (*Frieda's Sugarloaf*), 1 oz. 14
fresh, sliced (*Dole*), 2 slices 90

canned:
    in juice, crushed (*Dole*) 70
    in juice, chunks or tidbits (*Dole*) 60
    in juice, sliced (*Dole*), 4 oz., 2 slices 60
    in light syrup, all varieties, except sliced (*Dole*) 80
    in light syrup, sliced (*Dole*), 2 slices 90
    in heavy syrup, all varieties, except sliced (*Dole*) 90
    in heavy syrup, sliced (*Dole*), 4 oz., 2 slices 90
    in extra heavy syrup, crushed (*Dole*) 110
    in extra heavy syrup, cubes (*Dole*) 200
dried (*Sonoma*), 1.4 oz. 140
in jars, chunks (*Sunfresh*) 90
Pineapple, candied, slices (*S&W* Glace), 2.2 oz. 180
Pineapple drink blends:
coconut, nectar (*Kern's*), 8 fl. oz. 200
grapefruit, pink (*Dole*), 8 fl. oz. 130
guava, nectar (*Goya*), 12 fl. oz. 230
passion fruit, nectar (*Goya*), 12 fl. oz. 220
Pineapple juice, 8 fl. oz.:
(*Del Monte*) 130
(*S&W*) 110
chilled (*Dole*) 130
frozen* (*Minute Maid*) 130
Pineapple juice blends, 8 fl. oz.:
coconut (*R. W. Knudsen*) 130
grapefruit, frozen* (*Dole*) 130
orange, frozen* (*Minute Maid*) 120
orange or orange-guava (*Dole*) 120
orange-banana or orange-berry (*Dole*) 130
passion fruit–banana (*Dole*) 120
Pineapple topping (*Smucker's*), 2 tbsp. 110
Pink beans, boiled, 1/2 cup 125
Pinto beans:
dry (*Goya*), 1/4 cup 60
canned (*Goya*), 1/2 cup 80
canned (*Green Giant/Joan of Arc*), 1/2 cup 110
canned (*Old El Paso*), 1/2 cup 100
canned, in tomato sauce (*Goya* Guisadas), 1/2 cup 100
Pinto beans, sprouted, boiled, drained, 4 oz. 25

Pistachio nuts, shelled, except as noted:
dried (*Dole*), 1 oz. 163
dry-roasted, in shell (*Planters*), ½ cup, 1 oz. edible 160
dry-roasted (*Planters*), 1 oz. 160
Pita, see "Bread"
Pizza, frozen:
bacon burger (*Totino's Party*), ½ pie, 5.25 oz. 380
Canadian bacon (*Jeno's Crisp 'n Tasty*), 6.9-oz pie 430
Canadian bacon (*Tombstone* Original 12″), ¼ pie 360
cheese (*Amy's*), 1 serving 310
cheese (*Celeste* for One), 1 pie 540
cheese, extra (*Marie Callender's*), ½ pie, 4.5 oz. 410
cheese, extra (*Tombstone* Original 9″), ½ pie 420
cheese, extra (*Tombstone For One*), 1 pie 540
cheese, extra (*Weight Watchers*), 5.74 oz. 390
cheese, four (*Celeste* for One), 1 pie 540
cheese, four, hot and zesty (*Celeste* for One), 1 pie 530
cheese, three (*Pappalo's* Deep Dish for One),
    7.2-oz. pie 540
cheese, three (*Pappalo's* Pizzaria Style 9″), ½ pie 400
cheese, two:
    w/Canadian bacon (*Totino's* Select), ⅓ pie, 4.9 oz. . . 310
    w/pepperoni (*Totino's* Select), ⅓ pie, 4.8 oz. 360
    w/sausage (*Totino's* Select), ⅓ pie, 5 oz. 360
combination (*Totino's Party*), ½ pie, 3.4 oz. 390
combination (*Weight Watchers* Deluxe), 6.57 oz. 380
deluxe (*Celeste* for One), 1 pie 540
deluxe (*Tombstone* Original 9″), ⅓ pie 320
hamburger (*Jeno's Crisp 'n Tasty*), 7.3-oz. pie 500
hamburger (*Tombstone* Original 9″), ⅓ pie 310
w/meat (*Celeste* Suprema for One), 1 pie 580
meat, four (*Pappalo's* Pizzaria Style 12″), ¼ pie 380
meat, three (*Totino's Party*), ½ pie, 5.25 oz. 360
Mexican style, zesty (*Totino's Party*), ½ pie, 5.5 oz. 370
pepperoni (*Celeste* Pizza for One), 1 pie 520
pepperoni (*Marie Callender's*), ½ pie, 4.5 oz. 440
pepperoni (*Pappalo's* Deep Dish), ⅕ pie, 4.4 oz. 340
pepperoni (*Pappalo's* Pizzaria Style 9″), ½ pie 440
pepperoni (*Weight Watchers*), 5.56 oz. 390

pepperoni, double cheese (*Tombstone Double Top*),
⅙ pie, 4.6 oz. 350
sausage (*Celeste* for One), 1 pie 530
sausage (*Pappalo's* Deep Dish), ⅕ pie, 4.6 oz. 330
sausage (*Pappalo's* Pizzaria Style 9″), ½ pie 440
sausage (*Tombstone* Original 9″), ⅓ pie 310
sausage, double cheese (*Tombstone Double Top*), ⅙ pie,
4.8 oz. 350
sausage, Italian (*Tombstone For One*), 7-oz. pie 560
sausage/mushroom (*Tombstone* Original 12″), ⅕ pie . . . 320
sausage and pepperoni:
  (*Pappalo's* Deep Dish), ⅕ pie, 4.6 oz. 530
  (*Pappalo's* for One), 7.2-oz. pie 570
  (*Pappalo's* Pizzaria Style 9″), ½ pie 440
  (*Tombstone* Original 9″), ⅓ pie 360
  (*Tombstone For One*), 7-oz. pie 590
  double cheese (*Tombstone Double Top*), ⅙ pie,
  4.8 oz. 360
supreme (*Pappalo's* Deep Dish), ⅕ pie, 4.9 oz. 350
supreme (*Pappalo's* for One), 7.6-oz. pie 520
supreme (*Pappalo's* Pizzaria Style 9″), ½ pie 300
supreme (*Tombstone* Original 12″), ⅕ pie 330
supreme (*Tombstone* Light), ⅕ pie, 4.9 oz. 270
super (*Tombstone Special Order* 9″), ⅓ pie 400
tomato and mozzarella (*Marie Callender's*), ½ pie,
4.5 oz. 350
vegetable (*Celeste* for One), 1 pie 480
vegetable (*Tombstone* Light), ⅕ pie, 4.6 oz. 240
Pizza, bagel (*Empire* Kosher), 2-oz. piece 150
Pizza, croissant, frozen, 1 piece:
cheese (*Pepperidge Farm*) 390
deluxe (*Pepperidge Farm*) 450
pepperoni (*Pepperidge Farm*) 420
Pizza, English muffin (*Empire* Kosher), 2-oz. piece 130
Pizza, French bread, frozen:
bacon cheddar (*Stouffer's*), ½ of 11⅜-oz. pkg. 430
cheese (*Healthy Choice*), 6 oz. 320
cheese (*Lean Cuisine*), 6 oz. 320
cheese (*Stouffer's*), ½ of 10⅜-oz. pkg. 360
cheeseburger (*Stouffer's*), ½ of 11⅞-oz. pkg. 420

Pizza, French bread *(cont.)*
deluxe (*Lean Cuisine*), 6⅛ oz. 320
deluxe (*Stouffer's*), ½ of 12⅜-oz. pkg. 430
meat, three (*Stouffer's*), ½ of 12½-oz. pkg. 460
pepperoni (*Healthy Choice*), 6 oz. 340
pepperoni (*Lean Cuisine*), 5¼ oz. 310
pepperoni (*Stouffer's*), ½ of 11¼-oz. pkg. 440
pepperoni and mushroom (*Stouffer's*),
  ½ of 12¼-oz. pkg. 440
sausage (*Healthy Choice*), 6 oz. 300
sausage (*Stouffer's*), ½ of 12-oz. pkg. 430
sausage and pepperoni (*Stouffer's*),
  ½ of 12½-oz. pkg. 450
supreme (*Healthy Choice*), 6 oz. 310
vegetable (*Healthy Choice*), 6 oz. 270
vegetable, deluxe (*Stouffer's*), ½ of 12¾-oz. pkg. 380
white (*Stouffer's*), ½ of 10⅛-oz. pkg. 460
Pizza crust, refrigerated (*Totino's*), ¼ crust 180
Pizza crust mix* (*Ragú Pizza Quick*), ⅕ of 12″ crust . . . 130
Pizza snacks, 6 pieces:
cheese, three (*Totino's Pizza Rolls*) 200
combination (*Totino's Pizza Rolls*) 220
hamburger and cheese (*Totino's Pizza Rolls*) 200
Italian style, spicy (*Totino's Pizza Rolls*) 220
meat, three (*Totino's Pizza Rolls*) 210
pepperoni and cheese (*Totino's Pizza Rolls*) 230
sausage and cheese, supreme (*Totino's Pizza Rolls*) . . . 210
sausage and mushroom (*Totino's Pizza Rolls*) 200
Pizza sandwich, frozen:
meat, mega (*Totino's* Big & Hearty), 4.8-oz. piece 330
pepperoni (*Deli Stuffs*), 4.5-oz. piece 370
pepperoni (*Totino's* Big & Hearty), 4.8-oz. piece 350
Pizza sauce, ¼ cup:
(*Progresso*) 35
(*Ragú Pizza Quick 100% Natural*) 30
(*Ragú Pizza Quick Traditional*) 40
garlic and basil (*Ragú Pizza Quick*) 40
pepperoni (*Ragú Pizza Quick*) 60
tomato, chunky (*Ragú Pizza Quick*) 50
Pizza seasoning (*Tone's Presti's*), ¾ tsp. 10

Plantain, raw (*Frieda's*), 1 oz. 34
Plum:
fresh (*Dole*), 2 fruits 70
canned, in juice, ½ cup 73
canned, in light syrup, ½ cup 79
canned, in heavy syrup (*Comstock*), ½ cup 110
canned, in heavy syrup, whole (*S&W*), ½ cup 130
Plum sauce (*Ka-Me*), 2 tbsp. 80
Poi, ½ cup 134
Poke greens, canned (*Allens*), ½ cup 35
Polenta, 2 slices, ½":
(*San Gennaro*) 70
basil and garlic (*San Gennaro*) 71
sun-dried tomato (*San Gennaro*) 74
Polenta mix (*Fantastic Foods*), 1 cup* 260
Polish sausage (see also "Kielbasa"):
beef (*Hebrew National*), 3-oz. link 240
skinless (*John Morrell*), 2 oz. 180
Pollock, meat only, 4 oz.:
Atlantic, raw 104
Atlantic, baked, broiled, or microwaved 134
walleye, raw 91
walleye, baked, broiled, or microwaved 128
Pomegranate (*Dole*), 1 medium 104
Pomegranate juice (*R. W. Knudsen*), 8 fl. oz. 150
Pompano, Florida, meat only, 4 oz.:
raw 186
baked, broiled, or microwaved 239
Popcorn, unpopped, 3 tbsp., except as noted:
(*Arrowhead Mills*), ¼ cup, 1¾ oz. 180
microwave (*Smart Pop*), 2 tbsp. 100
microwave, butter (*Pop·Secret*) 180
microwave, butter (*Pop·Secret Movie Theater*) 170
microwave, butter, light (*Pop·Secret*) 140
microwave, butter, 94% fat free (*Pop·Secret*) 120
microwave, butter, real (*Pop·Secret*) 180
microwave, cheese, cheddar or nacho (*Pop·Secret*) . . . 180
microwave, natural (*Pop·Secret*) 170
microwave, natural, light (*Pop·Secret*) 140
microwave, natural, 94% fat free (*Pop·Secret*) 120

Popcorn, popped:
(*Wise* Choice), 2½ cups 140
air-popped (*Bachman*), 2¾ cups 170
air-popped (*Bachman* Lite), 5 cups 120
butter/butter flavor:
    (*Borden*), 1-oz. bag 150
    (*Smartfood*), 3 cups 150
    (*Smartfood* Reduced Fat), 3⅓ cups 130
    (*Wise* Reduced Fat), 3 cups 130
caramel:
    (*Cracker Jack* Fat Free), 1 cup, 1 oz. 110
    (*Smart Snackers*), .9-oz. bag 100
    (*Wise* Fat Free), 1 cup 110
    w/peanuts (*Cracker Jack*), ⅔ cup 120
    w/peanuts (*Cracker Jack*), 1.25-oz. box 150
cheddar, white (*Barrel O'Fun*), 3 cups 185
cheddar, white (*Smartfood* Reduced Fat), 3 cups 140
microwave, 1 cup:
    cheese, cheddar or nacho (*Pop·Secret*) 30
    natural (*Pop·Secret*) 35
    natural, light (*Pop·Secret*) 25
    natural, 94% fat free (*Pop·Secret*) 20
    butter flavor (*Pop·Secret*) 35
    butter flavor (*Pop·Secret Movie Theater*) 40
    light (*Pop·Secret/Pop·Secret Movie Theater*) 25
    94% fat free (*Pop·Secret*) 20
    real (*Pop·Secret*) 35
toffee, butter:
    (*Cracker Jack* Fat Free), 1 cup, 1 oz. 110
    w/peanuts (*Cracker Jack*), 1.25-oz. box 160
    w/pecans and almonds (*Cracker Jack*), 1 oz. 130
Popcorn bar, caramel or chocolate (*Pop·Secret*), 1 bar . . 70
Popcorn cakes:
butter (*Quaker* Mini), 6 cakes 50
cheddar, white (*Lundberg* Mini), 5 cakes 70
Poppy seed (*McCormick*), ¼ tsp. 4
Pork, meat only (see also "Ham"), 4 oz., except as
    noted:
loin, whole, braised, lean w/fat 417
loin, whole, braised, lean only 310

loin, whole, broiled, lean w/fat 392
loin, whole, broiled, lean only 291
loin, whole, roasted, lean w/fat 362
loin, whole, roasted, lean only 272
loin, blade, broiled, lean w/fat 446
loin, blade, broiled, lean only 340
loin, blade, roasted, lean w/fat 413
loin, blade, roasted, lean only 316
loin, center, broiled, lean w/fat 358
loin, center, broiled, lean only 262
loin, center, roasted, lean w/fat 346
loin, center, roasted, lean only 272
loin, center rib, braised, lean w/fat 416
loin, center rib, braised, lean only 314
loin, center rib, broiled, lean w/fat 389
loin, center rib, broiled, lean only 293
loin, center rib, roasted, lean w/fat 361
loin, center rib, roasted, lean only 278
loin, top, braised, lean w/fat 432
loin, top, braised, lean only 314
loin, top, broiled, lean w/fat 408
loin, top, broiled, lean only 293
loin, top, roasted, lean only 278
shoulder, whole, roasted, lean w/fat 370
shoulder, whole, roasted, lean only 277
shoulder, arm (picnic), roasted, lean w/fat 375
shoulder, arm (picnic), roasted, lean only 259
shoulder, Boston blade, braised, lean w/fat 421
shoulder, Boston blade, braised, lean only 333
shoulder, Boston blade, broiled, lean w/fat 397
shoulder, Boston blade, broiled, lean only 311
shoulder, Boston blade, roasted, lean only 290
sirloin, braised, lean w/fat 399
sirloin, braised, lean only 296
sirloin, broiled, lean w/fat 375
sirloin, broiled, lean only 276
sirloin, roasted, lean w/fat 330
sirloin, roasted, lean only 268
spareribs, braised, lean w/fat, 6.3 oz. (1 lb. raw
   w/bone) 703

Pork *(cont.)*
tenderloin, roasted, lean only 188
Pork, cured (see also "Ham"), 4 oz.:
arm (picnic), roasted, lean w/fat 318
arm (picnic), roasted, lean only 193
blade roll, lean w/fat, roasted 325
Pork batter, frying (*House of Tsang*), 4 tbsp. 140
Pork belly, raw, 1 oz. 147
Pork chow mein, canned (*La Choy* Bi-Pack), 1 cup 80
Pork dinner, frozen, 1 pkg.:
barbecue (*Swanson Hungry Man*) 770
patty, grilled glazed (*Healthy Choice*), 9.6 oz. 280
Pork entree, frozen:
rib-shape patty, barbecue (*Swanson*), 1 pkg. 460
sweet and sour (*Chun King*), 13 oz. 450
Pork gravy (*Heinz* Homestyle), 1/4 cup 25
Pork lunch meat, seasoned (*Boar's Head*), 2 oz. 80
Pork patty, frozen (*Tyson*), 3.8-oz. patty 200
Pork rind snack, 1/2 oz.:
(*Baken-ets/Baken-ets* Cracklins) 80
hot and spicy (*Baken-ets*) 70
hot and spicy (*Baken-ets* Cracklins) 80
Pork seasoning mix:
(*Durkee/French's* Roasting Bag), 1/6 pkg. 25
chops (*McCormick Bag 'n Season*), 2 tsp. mix 15
sparerib (*Durkee* Roasting Bag), 1/7 pkg. 25
Pork and beans, see "Baked beans"
Pot roast seasoning mix, 1/6 pkg.:
(*Durkee* Roasting Bag) 15
(*French's* Roasting Bag) 20
onion (*French's* Roasting Bag) 25
Potato:
(*Dole*), 1 medium, 5.3 oz. 100
baked in skin, 1 medium, 4 3/4" × 2 1/3" diam. 220
boiled in skin, baby (*Frieda's*), 4 oz. 86
boiled w/out skin, 2 1/2"-diam. potato 116
microwaved in skin, 1 medium, 4 3/4" × 2 1/3" diam. 212
mashed, w/whole milk, 1/2 cup 81
Potato, canned:
(*Seneca*), 2/3 cup 80

whole, new (*Del Monte*), 2 medium w/liquid 60
sliced (*Del Monte*), ²/₃ cup 60
mashed (*Idahoan* Real), ¹/₃ cup 80
Potato, frozen (see also "Potato dishes, frozen"):
whole (*Stilwell*), 3 pieces 50
(*Ore-Ida* Deep Fries/Deep Fries Crinkle Cuts), 3 oz. 160
(*Ore-Ida* Shoestrings), 3 oz. 150
(*Ore-Ida* Steak Fries), 3 oz. 110
(*Ore-Ida Crispers!*), 3 oz. 220
(*Ore-Ida Golden Crinkles*), 3 oz. 140
(*Ore-Ida Golden Fries*), 3 oz. 120
crinkle cut (*Empire* Kosher), ¹/₂ cup 90
hash brown (*Ore-Ida Golden Patties*), 1 piece 160
hash brown, w/cheddar (*Ore-Ida Cheddar Browns*),
    1 piece 80
mashed (*Ore-Ida*), ²/₃ cup 90
O'Brien (*Ore-Ida*), ³/₄ cup 60
puffs (*Hot Tots/Tater Tots*), 3 oz. 160
Potato, mix*:
(*Betty Crocker Potato Shakers*), ²/₃ cup 140
(*Betty Crocker Potato Buds*), ²/₃ cup 160
au gratin or broccoli (*Betty Crocker*), ¹/₂ cup 110
broccoli, stove-top recipe (*Betty Crocker*), ¹/₂ cup 130
cheddar (*Betty Crocker/Betty Crocker Cheddar &
    Bac·Os*), ¹/₂ cup 120
cheddar (*Betty Crocker Potato Buds*), ²/₃ cup 190
cheddar, zesty (*Betty Crocker Potato Shakers*), ²/₃ cup . . 140
cheddar and bacon (*Betty Crocker* Twice Baked),
    ²/₃ cup 210
cheddar and sour cream (*Betty Crocker*), ¹/₂ cup 130
cheese, Parmesan, and herb (*Betty Crocker Potato
    Shakers*), ²/₃ cup 140
cheese, three (*Betty Crocker*), ¹/₂ cup 120
fries, seasoned (*Betty Crocker Potato Shakers*),
    7 fries 120
garlic (*Betty Crocker Potato Shakers*), ²/₃ cup 130
hash brown (*Betty Crocker*), ¹/₂ cup 200
julienne (*Betty Crocker*), ¹/₂ cup 110
mashed, all flavors (*Hungry Jack*), ¹/₂ cup 150
ranch or scalloped (*Betty Crocker*), ¹/₂ cup 130

Potato, mix *(cont.)*

scalloped, cheesy or w/ham (*Betty Crocker*), ½ cup . . . 120
sour cream and chive (*Betty Crocker*), ½ cup 120
Potato cheddar pocket (*Ken & Robert's Veggie Pockets*),
  1 piece 260
Potato chips and crisps, 1 oz.:

(*Kettle* Chips) 150
(*Kettle* Crisps) 110
(*Lay's/Lay's* Unsalted) 150
(*Pringles* Original) 160
(*Wise* Ripple) 150
all varieties (*Lay's* Baked) 110
all varieties (*Lay's* Wavy) 160
all varieties (*Pringles* Ridges) 150
all varieties (*Pringles Right Crisps*) 140
barbecue (*Lay's* Hickory/*Lay's KC Masterpiece*) 150
barbecue, honey (*Kettle* Crisps) 110
Caribbean flavor (*Borden* Calypso) 160
cheddar, New York, w/herbs (*Kettle* Chips) 150
cheddar and sour cream (*Wise*) 150
cheese (*Pringles Cheez Ums*) 150
honey Dijon (*Kettle* Chips) 150
hot (*Lay's* Flamin') 150
jalapeño jack (*Kettle* Chips) 140
onion and garlic (*Borden*) 150
onion and garlic (*Lay's*) 150
pesto (*Kettle* Crisps) 110
ranch (*Pringles*) 150
salsa and cheese (*Lay's*) 160
salsa w/mesquite (*Kettle* Chips) 140
salt and vinegar (*Borden*) 150
salt and vinegar (*Kettle* Chips) 150
sour cream and onion or salt and vinegar (*Lay's*) 160
sour cream and onion (*Borden*) 150
sour cream and onion (*Pringles*) 160
yogurt and green onion (*Kettle* Chips) 150
Potato dishes, canned, 7.5 oz.:

au gratin, and bacon (*Hormel*) 250
scalloped, and ham (*Nalley*) 210
sliced, and beef (*Dinty Moore*) 230

Potato dishes, frozen:
(*Goya* Rellenos de Papa), 2 pieces 280
au gratin (*Stouffer's* Side Dish), 4.6 oz. 130
baked, butter flavor (*Ore-Ida* Twice Baked), 5 oz. 200
baked, broccoli and cheese (*Weight Watchers*), 10 oz. . . 250
baked, cheddar (*Ore-Ida* Twice Baked), 5 oz. 190
baked, sour cream/chive (*Ore-Ida* Twice Baked), 5 oz. . . 200
cheddar broccoli (*Healthy Choice*), 1 pkg. 310
garden casserole (*Healthy Choice*), 1 pkg. 210
mozzarella, w/chicken (*The Budget Gourmet* Italian
  Originals), 10.13 oz. 390
roasted, w/broccoli, cheese sauce (*Lean Cuisine Lunch
  Classics*), 1 pkg. 210
Potato flour, 1 cup 628
Potato pancake, frozen (*Empire* Kosher), 2-oz. cake . . . 80
Potato pancake mix* (*Hungry Jack*), 3 cakes, 3″ 90
Potato salad seasoning (*Tone's*), 1 tsp. 5
Potato sticks:
(*French's*), 1 cup 250
shoestring (*Pik-Nik*), ²/₃ cup 160
shoestring, BBQ or sour cream/cheddar (*Pik-Nik*),
  ²/₃ cup 180
Potpie, see specific entree listings
Poultry, see specific listings
Poultry seasoning, 1 tsp. 5
Pout, ocean, meat only, 4 oz.:
raw 90
baked, broiled, or microwaved 116
Preserves, see "Jam and preserves"
Pretzels:
(*Bachman* Fat Free Thins), 11 pieces 110
(*Bachman* Twist/Butter Twist), 5 pieces 110
(*Barbara's* Honeysweet), 1 oz. 100
(*Borden* Thins/Tiny Thins/Mini/Ultra Thins), 1 oz. 100
(*Thin 'n Right*), 12 pieces 120
all varieties (*Combos*), 1 oz. 130
nuggets (*Nutzels*), ¹/₂ cup 110
rods (*Bachman*), 2 pieces 110
sticks (*Bachman Stix*), 1 oz. 100
Pretzel dip (*Nance's*), 2 tbsp. 90

Prickly pear (*Frieda's*), 3½ oz. 42
Prosciutto (*Primissimo*), 2 oz. 210
Prune:
canned, in heavy syrup, stewed (*S&W*), 8 pieces,
    4.9 oz. 210
dried (*Del Monte*), ¼ cup 120
dried, pitted (*Sonoma*), ¼ cup 120
Prune juice (*Del Monte*), 8 fl. oz. 170
Pudding, 4 oz., except as noted:
banana (*Thank You*), ½ cup 200
banana, nondairy (*Imagine*) 150
butterscotch (*Thank You*), ½ cup 160
butterscotch, nondairy (*Imagine*) 150
chocolate (*Jell-O* Snack) 160
chocolate (*Jell-O Free* Snack) 100
chocolate (*Thank You*), ½ cup 190
chocolate, nondairy (*Imagine*) 170
chocolate swirl, caramel or vanilla (*Jell-O* Snack) . . 160
chocolate swirl, caramel or vanilla (*Jell-O Free* Snack) . . 100
lemon, nondairy (*Imagine*) 150
tapioca (*Thank You*), ½ cup 160
vanilla (*Jell-O Free* Snack) 100
vanilla (*Thank You*), ½ cup 160
vanilla-chocolate swirl (*Jell-O Snack)* 170
vanilla-chocolate swirl (*Jell-O Free* Snack) 100
Pudding mix*, ½ cup:
banana (*Jell-O* Sugar/Fat Free) 70
banana cream (*Jell-O*) 140
banana cream (*Jell-O* Instant) 150
butter pecan (*Jell-O* Instant) 160
butterscotch (*Jell-O*) 160
butterscotch (*Jell-O* Instant) 150
butterscotch (*Jell-O* Sugar/Fat Free) 70
chocolate (*D-Zerta*) 60
chocolate, all flavors (*Jell-O*) 150
chocolate, all flavors (*Jell-O* Instant) 160
chocolate, all flavors (*Jell-O* Sugar/Fat Free) 80
chocolate (*My*T*Fine*) 90
coconut cream (*Jell-O*) 150
coconut cream (*Jell-O* Instant) 160

custard (*Jell-O Americana*) 140
custard, tropical (*Goya* Tembleque) 100
flan (*Goya*) 100
flan (*Jell-O*) 140
flan, w/caramel (*Goya*) 190
lemon (*Jell-O*) 140
lemon (*Jell-O* Instant) 150
pistachio (*Jell-O* Instant) 160
pistachio (*Jell-O* Sugar/Fat Free) 70
rice, see "Rice pudding mix"
tapioca (*Jell-O Americana*) 140
vanilla (*Jell-O*) 140
vanilla (*Jell-O* Instant) 160
vanilla (*Jell-O* Sugar Free) 80
vanilla (*Jell-O* Sugar/Fat Free) 70
vanilla, French (*Jell-O* Instant) 150
Pummelo (*Frieda's*), 3.5 oz. 38
Pumpkin, canned, ½ cup:
fresh, pulp, boiled, drained, mashed 24
canned (*Comstock*) 50
canned (*Libby's*) 60
pie mix, see "Pie filling"
Pumpkin pie spice, 1 tsp. 6
Pumpkin seeds:
roasted, in shell, salted or unsalted, 85 seeds, 1 oz. . . . 127
roasted, shelled, salted or unsalted, 1 oz. 148
tamari-roasted, spicy (*Eden*), 1 oz. 170

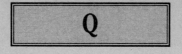

Q

FOOD AND MEASURE **CALORIES**

Quail, raw:
meat w/skin, 1 quail, 3.8 oz. (4.3 oz. w/bone) 210
meat w/skin, 1 oz. 54
meat only, 1 quail, 3.2 oz. (4.3 oz. w/bone and skin) . . . 123
meat only, 1 oz. 38
breast meat only, 1 breast, 2 oz. 69
breast meat only, 1 oz. 35
Quince, 1 medium, 5.3 oz. 53
Quincy's Family Steakhouse:
breakfast items:
   apples, escalloped, 3.5 oz. 120
   bacon, ¼ oz. 35
   corned beef hash, 4.5 oz. 210
   eggs, scrambled, 2 oz. 95
   ham, 1.5 oz. 90
   oatmeal, 1 oz. 175
   pancakes, 1.5 oz. 95
   sausage gravy, 4 oz. 70
   sausage links, 2 oz. 225
   sausage patties, 2 oz. 230
   steak fingers, 3.5 oz. 360
   syrup, 1 oz. 75
beef entrees:
   fillet w/bacon, 8 oz. before cooking 340
   sirloin tips w/pepper and onions, 5 oz. 203
   sirloin tips w/mushroom gravy, 6 oz. 196
   steak, chopped, 8 oz. before cooking 499
   steak, country, w/gravy, 9 oz. 530
   steak, cowboy, 14 oz. before cooking 580
   steak, New York strip, 10 oz. 450
   steak, porterhouse, 17 oz. before cooking 683
   steak, ribeye, 10 oz. before cooking 452
   steak, sirloin, junior, 5.5 oz. before cooking 194

steak, sirloin, regular, 8 oz. before cooking 285
steak, sirloin, large, 10 oz. before cooking 368
steak, strip, smothered, 10 oz. before cooking 622
steak, T-bone, 13 oz. before cooking 521
other entree items:
chicken, grilled, 5 oz. 120
chicken fillet, homestyle, 3 oz. 217
chicken, roasted, w/herbs, 14 oz. 875
chicken, roasted BBQ, 14 oz. 941
salmon, grilled, 7 oz. 228
shrimp, breaded, 7 oz. 546
steak and shrimp, 9 oz. 677
sandwiches, 1 piece:
burger, 1/3 pound 565
burger, bacon cheese 663
chicken, grilled 324
chicken, spicy BBQ 368
steak, Philly cheese 588
steak, smothered 429
side dishes, 4 oz., except as noted:
apples, w/cinnamon 172
beans, BBQ 114
beans, green 61
broccoli spears 34
broccoli spears, w/cheese sauce, 5 oz. 92
corn 96
potatoes, baked, plain, 6 oz. 115
potatoes, mashed 54
potatoes, steak fries 358
rice pilaf 119
bread, 2 oz.:
banana nut 165
biscuit 270
corn bread 140
roll, yeast 160
soups, 6 oz.:
broccoli, cream of 170
chili 235
clam chowder 180
vegetable beef 90

Quincy's Family Steakhouse (cont.)
salad dressings, 1 oz.:

    bleu cheese 155
    French 125
    French, light 85
    honey mustard 100
    Italian 135
    Italian, light 20
    Italian, light, creamy 65
    Parmesan peppercorn 150
    ranch 110
    Thousand Island, light 65
desserts:
    brownie pudding cake, 4 oz. 310
    cobbler, apple, 6 oz. 255
    cobbler, cherry, 6 oz. 410
    cobbler, peach, 6 oz. 305
    cookie, chocolate chip or sugar, 1/2 oz. 60
    pudding, banana, 5 oz. 240
    yogurt, frozen, 4 oz. 135
    yogurt toppings, caramel or fudge, 1 oz. 105
Quinoa:
(*Eden*), 1/4 cup 170
black and white (*Frieda's*), 2 oz. dry or 1/2 cup cooked . . 218
Quinoa seeds (*Arrowhead Mills*), 1/4 cup 140

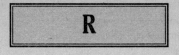

R

FOOD AND MEASURE   **CALORIES**

Rabbit, domesticated, 4 oz.:
meat only, roasted 223
meat only, stewed 234
Radiatore entree, frozen (*Hain* Bolognese), 10 oz. 290
Radicchio, fresh, shredded, ½ cup 5
Radish (*Dole*), 7 pieces 20
Radish, Oriental, raw, sliced, ½ cup 8
Radish, white-icicle, raw, sliced, ½ cup 7
Radish sprouts (*Jonathan's*), 1 cup 57
Rainbow baking morsels (*Nestlé*), 1 tbsp. 70
Raisins, seedless, golden seedless, or muscat
   (*Sun·Maid*), ¼ cup 130
Ranch dip, 2 tbsp.:
(*Kraft*) 60
(*Marie's* Creamy) 190
(*Marie's* Homestyle) 150
vegetable (*Bernstein's*) 120
Raspberry:
fresh (*Dole*), 3 oz. 40
canned, in heavy syrup (*Comstock*), ½ cup 100
frozen, red (*Birdseye*), ½ cup 90
Raspberry juice, 8 fl. oz.:
blend (*Dole* Country) 140
cranberry (*Apple & Eve*) 120
Raspberry nectar (*Santa Cruz*), 8 fl. oz. 100
Raspberry syrup (*R. W. Knudsen*), ¼ cup 150
Ravioli, frozen or refrigerated:
beef and garlic (*Contadina*), 1¼ cups 350
cheese (*Amy's*), 9.5 oz. 340
cheese (*Celentano*), ½ of 13-oz. pkg. 400
cheese (*Contadina* Family Pack), 1 cup 290
cheese, four (*Contadina* Light), 1 cup 240
cheese and garlic (*Di Giorno* Light), 1 cup 270

Ravioli *(cont.)*

chicken, rosemary (*Contadina*), 1¼ cups 330
garden vegetable (*Contadina* Light), 1 cup 250
Gorgonzola (*Contadina*), 1¼ cups 360
w/Italian sausage (*Di Giorno*), ¾ cup 340
tofu (*Tofutti*), 1 cup 320
tomato and cheese (*Di Giorno* Light), 1 cup 280

Ravioli entree, canned, 1 cup:

w/beef, tomato sauce (*Hunt's* Homestyle) 220
w/beef, tomato sauce (*Nalley*) 280
w/beef, tomato sauce (*Progresso*) 260
w/cheese, tomato sauce (*Progresso*) 220

Ravioli entree, frozen, 1 pkg.:

cheese (*Stouffer's*), 10⅝ oz. 380
Florentine (*Smart Ones*), 8.5 oz. 220
mushroom and spinach (*Wolfgang Puck's*), 13 oz. 260
parmigiana (*Healthy Choice*), 9 oz. 260

Red beans, canned:

(*Goya*), ¼ cup 160
(*Green Giant/Joan of Arc*), ½ cup 100

Red bean dish mix:

New Orleans (*Fantastic* One Pot Meals), ½ cup 150
w/radiatore (*Bean Cuisine* Barcelona), ½ cup* 170

Red snapper, see "Snapper"
Redfish, see "Ocean perch"

Refried beans, canned, ½ cup:

(*Gebhardt*) 110
(*Gebhardt* No Fat) 90
(*Goya*) 110
(*Old El Paso*) 110
all varieties (*Old El Paso* Fat Free) 100
black beans (*Old El Paso*) 110
w/cheese (*Old El Paso*) 130
w/green chilies (*Old El Paso*) 100
w/jalapeño (*Gebhardt*) 105
w/sausage (*Old El Paso*) 200
spicy (*Old El Paso*) 140
vegetarian (*Old El Paso*) 100

Refried beans, mix (*Fantastic Foods* Instant), ½ cup* . . 160
Relish, see "Pickle relish" and specific listings

Rhubarb:
fresh, regular or hothouse (*Frieda's*), 1 oz. 5
frozen (*Stilwell*), 1 cup 30
Rice (see also "Wild rice"), dry, ¼ cup, except as noted:
Arborio (*Frieda's*) 210
basmati, brown (*Lundberg* Organic) 160
basmati, brown (*Lundberg Nutra-Farmed*/Royal) 170
basmati, white (*Lundberg Nutra-Farmed*/Organic) 180
blends (*Lundberg Countrywild/Wild Blend*) 150
blends (*Lundberg Jubilee/Black Japonica*) 170
brown (*Carolina/Mahatma/River*) 150
brown (*Lundberg Wehani*) 170
brown, long or short grain (*Lundberg Nutra-Farmed/*
    Organic) 170
brown, long grain (*Uncle Ben's* Whole Grain) 170
brown, medium grain (*Lundberg*) 160
brown, quick or sweet (*Lundberg*) 150
glutinous or sweet (*Goya* Blue Rose/Valencia) 170
white, long grain (*Carolina*) 150
white, extra long grain (*Goya*) 160
instant (*Carolina*) 160
instant (*Minute*), ½ cup 170
instant (*Minute* Boil-in-Bag), ½ cup 190
Rice cakes, all varieties (*Lundberg*), 1 cake 60
Rice chips, brown (*Eden*), 50 chips, 1.1 oz. 150
Rice dishes, canned:
Chinese fried (*La Choy*), 1 cup 240
Mexican (*Old El Paso*), ½ cup 410
Spanish (*Old El Paso*), 1 cup 130
Rice dishes, frozen (see also "Rice entree, frozen"):
and broccoli (*Green Giant*), 1 pkg. 320
and broccoli, au gratin (*Freezer Queen* Side Dish), 1 cup 180
and vegetables:
    (*Green Giant* Medley), 1 pkg. 240
    Oriental (*Green Giant* International), 1 pkg. 180
    pilaf (*Green Giant*), 1 pkg. 230
    white and wild (*Green Giant*), 1 pkg. 250
Rice dishes, mix, 2 oz. dry, except as noted:
and beans, black (*Carolina/Mahatma*) 200
and beans, black or red (*Goya*) 160

Rice dishes, mix *(cont.)*

and beans, black, Mediterranean, pilaf *(Near East)* 270
and beans, red *(Rice-A-Roni)*, 1 cup* 280
beef *(Rice-A-Roni)*, 1 cup* 320
beef and mushroom *(Rice-A-Roni)*, 1 cup* 290
broccoli au gratin *(Rice-A-Roni)*, 1 cup* 370
cheddar, white, w/herbs *(Rice-A-Roni)*, 1 cup* 340
chicken *(Rice-A-Roni)*, 1 cup* 310
chicken and broccoli *(Rice-A-Roni)*, 1 cup* 290
chicken and mushrooms *(Rice-A-Roni)*, 1 cup* 360
chicken w/vegetables *(Rice-A-Roni)*, 1 cup* 290
curry, basmati, w/lentils *(Fantastic* One Pot Meals),
   ³/₈ cup 160
fried *(Rice-A-Roni)*, 1 cup* 320
herb and butter *(Rice-A-Roni)*, 1 cup* 310
jambalaya *(Mahatma)* 190
long grain and wild *(Rice-A-Roni)*, 1 cup* 240
long grain and wild, chicken w/almonds *(Rice-A-Roni)*,
   1 cup* 290
long grain and wild, pilaf *(Rice-A-Roni)*, 1 cup* 240
Mexican *(Goya)*, ¼ cup 160
Mexican, cheesy *(Old El Paso)*, ½ pkg. 420
Oriental *(Rice-A-Roni)*, 1 cup* 290
pilaf *(Casbah)*, 1 oz. 100
pilaf *(Rice-A-Roni)*, 1 cup* 310
pilaf, brown rice, w/miso *(Fantastic Foods)*, ½ cup 250
pilaf, 4 grain w/wild rice *(Fantastic* Healthy
   Complements), ½ cup 160
pilaf, 3 grain w/herbs *(Fantastic Foods)*, ⅓ cup 240
risotto, all varieties *(Lundberg)*, ¼ pkg. 140
risotto, classico or mushroom *(Fantastic* Healthy
   Complements), ¼ cup 140
Spanish *(Fantastic* Healthy Complements), ³/₈ cup 160
Spanish *(Rice-A-Roni)*, 1 cup* 270
Spanish, brown rice pilaf *(Fantastic Foods)*, ½ cup 240
Spanish pilaf *(Casbah)*, 1 oz. 100
Stroganoff *(Rice-A-Roni)*, 1 cup* 360
yellow *(Goya)*, ¼ cup 170
yellow, saffron *(Carolina/Mahatma)* 190

Rice entree, frozen (see also "Rice dishes, frozen"):
and beans, Santa Fe (*Weight Watchers* International
   Selections), 10 oz. 290
cheese, four, w/pasta and chicken (*The Budget Gourmet*
   Italian Originals), 10.5 oz. 330
fried, w/chicken (*Chun King*), 8 oz. 270
fried, w/pork (*Chun King*), 8 oz. 290
Italian style, and chicken and mozzarella (*The Budget
   Gourmet* Italian Originals), 10 oz. 270
pilaf Florentine (*Weight Watchers* International
   Selections), 10.13 oz. 290
risotto, w/cheese, mushrooms (*Weight Watchers*),
   10 oz. 290
and vegetables, 1 pkg.:
   Hunan style (*Weight Watchers* International
     Selections) 250
   paella (*Weight Watchers* International Selections) . . . 280
   Peking style (*Weight Watchers* International
     Selections) 270
   stir-fry (*The Budget Gourmet* Value Classics) 410
   Szechuan, and chicken (*Smart Ones*) 220
wild, pilaf, (*The Budget Gourmet* Value Classics),
   8.5 oz. 400
Rice flour (*Goya*), 3 tbsp. 120
Rice pudding, canned (*Thank You*), ½ cup 160
Rice pudding mix:
(*Jell-O Americana*), ½ cup* 160
all varieties (*Lundberg* Elegant), ½ cup dry 70
Rice puffs, five flavor (*Eden*), 30 puffs, 1.1 oz. 110
Rice seasoning mix:
fried (*Durkee*), ¼ pkg. 15
Mexican (*Lawry's*), 1½ tbsp. 40
Rice syrup (*Lundberg Nutra-Farmed*/Organic), ¼ cup . . . 170
Rigatoni dishes, mix, approx. 1 cup*:
cheddar and broccoli (*Pasta Roni*) 400
tomato basil (*Pasta Roni*) 240
Rigatoni entree, frozen:
(*Freezer Queen* Family), 1 cup, 8.3 oz. 250
cream sauce, w/broccoli and chicken (*The Budget
   Gourmet* Special Selections), 9 oz. 230

Rigatoni entree, frozen *(cont.)*

creamy, w/broccoli and chicken (*Smart Ones*), 9 oz. . . . 230
parmigiana (*Marie Callender's*), 1 cup, 7.5 oz. 300
Rockfish, meat only, 4 oz.:
raw 107
baked, broiled, or microwaved 137
Roe (see also "Caviar"), raw, 1 tbsp. 22
Roll (see also "Biscuit"), 1 roll, except as noted:
(*Arnold Francisco 3"*) 90
(*Arnold Bran'nola* Buns) 130
assorted (*Brownberry* Hearth) 120
brown and serve (*Roman Meal*), 2 rolls 140
brown and serve (*Wonder* 12 oz.) 70
brown and serve, sourdough (*Arnold Francisco*) 80
dinner (*Arnold* 12 Pack/24 Pack) 110
dinner (*Arnold Bran'nola*) 70
dinner (*Roman Meal*), 2 rolls 150
dinner, potato or sesame seed (*Arnold*), 2 rolls 110
dinner, wheat (*Arnold August Bros.*) 100
dinner, white (*Arnold August Bros.*) 90
egg, twist (*Arnold Levy* Old Country) 170
French (*Arnold 6"*) 160
French, mini (*Arnold Francisco*) 110
hamburger (*Arnold* 8 Pack) 130
hamburger (*Roman Meal*) 120
hamburger (*Wonder*) 110
hot dog (*Arnold* 12 oz./12 Pack) 110
hot dog (*Wonder*) 110
Italian (*Arnold Savoni 8"*) 280
kaiser (*Arnold August Bros.*) 160
kaiser, sesame (*Arnold* Sandwich) 140
onion (*Arnold* Deli) 170
potato, plain or w/sesame (*Arnold*) 150
sandwich (*Roman Meal*) 185
sandwich, sesame, soft (*Arnold*) 140
sesame (*Arnold August Bros.*) 170
sourdough (*Arnold Francisco*) 90
sub (*Arnold August Bros.*) 170
tea (*Wonder*) 80

Roll, mix, hot:

(*Dromedary*), 1/16 pkg. 100

(*Pillsbury*), 1/15 pkg.* 130

Roll, refrigerated, crescent or dinner (*Pillsbury*), 1 roll   110

Roll, sweet, see "Bun, sweet"

Roman beans, canned (*Goya*), 1/4 cup 90

Rose apple, trimmed, 1 oz. 7

Rosemary, dried (*McCormick*), 1/4 tsp. 2

Roughy, orange, meat only, 4 oz.:

raw 143

baked, broiled, or microwaved 101

Rum runner mixer, raspberry, frozen* (*Bacardi*), 8 fl. oz. 120

Rutabaga, 1/2 cup:

fresh, boiled, drained, mashed 47

canned (*Sunshine*) 30

Rye, whole grain (*Arrowhead Mills*), 1/4 cup 160

Rye flakes, rolled (*Arrowhead Mills*), 1/3 cup 110

Rye flour:

(*Arrowhead Mills*), 1/4 cup 100

medium (*Pillsbury*), 1/4 cup 100

Rye-wheat flour (*Pillsbury* Bohemian Style), 1/4 cup 100

S

Sablefish, meat only, 4 oz.:
raw 222
baked, broiled, or microwaved 284
smoked 291
Salad, fresh, w/dressing, 3.5 oz., except as noted:
all varieties, except herb ranch (*Dole* Complete Lowfat) . 60
Caesar (*Dole* Complete) 170
Caesar (*Dole Lunch for One*), 5.75 oz. 300
Caesar (*Dole Lunch for One* Lowfat), 6 oz. 120
herb ranch (*Dole* Complete Lowfat) 50
Italian (*Dole Lunch for One* Lowfat), 7 oz. 110
Oriental (*Dole* Complete) 120
ranch (*Dole Lunch for One*), 7 oz. 340
Romano (*Dole* Complete) 150
spinach bacon (*Dole* Complete) 160
sunflower ranch (*Dole* Complete) 170
Salad blend mix, fresh, 3 oz.:
all varieties, except French (*Dole* Special Blends) 15
French (*Dole* Special Blends) 20
Salad dressing, 2 tbsp.:
bacon and tomato (*Kraft*) 140
bacon and tomato (*Kraft Deliciously Right*) 60
balsamic vinegar (*S&W* Vintage) 35
berry vinaigrette (*Knott's Berry Farm*) 40
blue cheese (*Bernstein's* Dressing/Dip) 180
blue cheese (*Bernstein's* Dressing/Dip Lite) 80
blue cheese (*Hellmann's*) 140
blue cheese (*Kraft Free*) 50
blue cheese (*Kraft Roka*) 90
blue cheese, chunky (*Seven Seas*) 90
blue cheese, creamy (*Bernstein's*) 120
Caesar (*Bernstein's*) 100
Caesar (*Bernstein's* Extra Rich) 110

Caesar (*Kraft*) 130
Caesar (*Kraft Deliciously Right*) 60
Caesar, creamy (*Hellmann's*) 170
cheese (*Bernstein's* Fantastico!) 110
cheese (*Bernstein's Light Fantastic* Fantastico!) 30
cheese (*Kraft*) 150
Dijon, creamy (*Bernstein's Light Fantastic*) 50
dill, creamy (*Bernstein's Light Fantastic*) 45
French (*Hellmann's* Fat Free) 45
French (*Kraft*) 120
French (*Kraft Catalina*) 140
French (*Kraft Deliciously Right*) 50
French (*Kraft Deliciously Right Catalina*) 80
French (*Kraft Free*) 50
French (*Kraft Free Catalina*) 45
French, herbal, creamy (*Bernstein's*) 130
French, w/honey (*Kraft Catalina*) 140
garden, zesty (*Kraft Salsa*) 70
garlic, creamy (*Kraft*) 110
green goddess (*Seven Seas*) 120
honey Dijon (*Hellmann's* Fat Free) 50
honey Dijon (*Kraft*) 150
honey Dijon (*Kraft Free*) 50
honey mustard (*Bernstein's* Dressing/Dip) 130
Italian (*Bernstein's*) 140
Italian (*Bernstein's* Reduced Calorie) 25
Italian (*Bernstein's* Restaurant) 80
Italian (*Bernstein's* Wine Country) 110
Italian (*Hellmann's*) 110
Italian (*Kraft* House) 120
Italian (*Kraft* Presto) 140
Italian (*Kraft Free*) 10
Italian, cheese and garlic (*Bernstein's*) 110
Italian, creamy (*Hellmann's*) 160
Italian, creamy (*Kraft*) 110
Italian, herb and garlic, creamy (*Bernstein's*) 130
Italian, zesty (*Kraft*) 110
mayonnaise type, see "Mayonnaise"
Oriental (*Bernstein's Light Fantastic*) 60
potato salad (*Best Foods/Hellmann's One Step*) 160

Salad dressing *(cont.)*
ranch (*Bernstein's* Dressing/Dip) 110
ranch (*Bernstein's* Dressing/Dip Lite) 70
ranch (*Bernstein's Light Fantastic*) 35
ranch (*Hellmann's* Fat Free) 45
ranch (*Hidden Valley* Original) 140
ranch (*Kraft*) 170
ranch (*Kraft Free*) 50
ranch (*Kraft Salsa*) 130
ranch (*Nalley*) 100
ranch (*Nalley* Fat Free) 40
ranch, buttermilk (*Kraft*) 150
ranch, creamy (*Hellmann's*) 140
ranch, cucumber (*Kraft*) 150
ranch, Italian (*Bernstein's*) 150
ranch, Parmesan garlic (*Bernstein's*) 110
ranch, Parmesan garlic (*Bernstein's Light Fantastic*) 45
ranch, peppercorn (*Kraft*) 170
ranch, peppercorn (*Kraft Free*) 50
ranch, sour cream and onion (*Kraft*) 170
red wine vinegar (*Kraft Free*) 15
Roquefort (*Bernstein's* Dressing/Dip) 140
Russian (*Kraft*) 130
salsa and sour cream (*Bernstein's* Dressing/Dip) 90
Thousand Island (*Bernstein's* Dressing/Dip) 120
Thousand Island (*Kraft*) 110
Thousand Island (*Kraft Free*) 45
Thousand Island (*Nalley*) 120
Thousand Island (*Nalley* Fat Free) 30
Thousand Island, w/bacon (*Kraft*) 120
tuna salad (*Best Foods/Hellmann's One Step*) 140
Salami, 2 oz., except as noted:
beef (*Boar's Head* Chub) 120
beef (*Hebrew National*) 170
beef (*Hebrew National* Reduced Fat) 110
dry or hard (*Boar's Head*), 1 oz. 110
Genoa (*Boar's Head*) 180
Genoa or hard (*Oscar Mayer*), 3 slices, 1 oz. 100
"Salami," vegetarian, frozen (*Worthington*), 3 slices . . 130

Salmon, fresh, meat only, 4 oz.:
Atlantic, farmed, raw 207
Atlantic, farmed, baked, broiled, or microwaved 234
Atlantic, wild, raw 161
Atlantic, wild, baked, broiled, or microwaved 206
chinook, raw 204
chinook, baked, broiled, or microwaved 262
chum, raw 136
chum, baked, broiled, or microwaved 175
coho, farmed, raw 182
coho, farmed, baked, broiled, or microwaved 202
coho, wild, raw 165
coho, wild, baked, broiled, or microwaved 158
coho, wild, boiled, poached, or steamed 209
pink, raw 132
pink, baked, broiled, or microwaved 169
sockeye, raw 191
sockeye, baked, broiled, or microwaved 245
Salmon, canned, ¼ cup:
pink, skinless fillet (*Bumble Bee*) 70
red (*Bumble Bee*) 110
red (*Libby's*) 110
Salmon, smoked:
chinook, 4 oz. 133
chinook, lox, 4 oz. 133
lox, Nova (*Vita*), 2 oz. 50
lox, Nova (*Vita*), 3-oz. pkg. 80
Salsa, 2 tbsp.:
(*Gracias*) 15
(*La Victoria* Ranchera) 10
(*La Victoria* Victoria) 5
all varieties (*Clemente Jacques*) 10
all varieties (*Nalley* Superba) 10
all varieties (*Old El Paso* Homestyle) 10
all varieties (*Old El Paso* Thick 'n Chunky) 15
all varieties (*Pace* Thick & Chunky) 10
all varieties (*Sun-Vista*) 5
all varieties except mild (*Las Palmas* Mexicana) 10
all varieties except verde (*Chi-Chi's*) 10
green or salsa verde (*Old El Paso*) 10

176 *Corinne T. Netzer*

Salsa *(cont.)*
mild (*Las Palmas* Mexicana) 5
verde, medium or mild (*Chi-Chi's*) 15
Salsify, raw, sliced, ½ cup 55
Salt pork, raw, 1 oz. 212
Sandwich sauce:
(*Durkee Famous*), 1 tbsp. 60
(*Manwich* Original), ¼ cup 30
barbecue or bold (*Manwich*), ¼ cup 60
Sloppy Joe (*Hormel Not-So-Sloppy Joe* Sauce), ¼ cup . . 70
Sloppy Joe (*Libby's*), ⅓ cup 45
Sandwich spread:
(*Hellmann's*), 1 tbsp. 50
(*Kraft* Spread & Burger Sauce), 1 tbsp. 50
(*Loma Linda*), ¼ cup 80
Sapodilla, ½ cup 100
Sapote, white (*Frieda's*), 1 oz. 35
Sardine, fresh, see "Herring"
Sardine, canned:
in lemon or spiced (*Goya*), ¼ cup 120
in mustard sauce (*Underwood*), 3¾-oz. can 180
in olive oil, drained (*Goya*), ¼ cup 130
in olive oil, drained (*Granadaisa*), ¼ cup 120
in olive oil, drained, small (*Goya* Sardinilla), ¼ cup 120
in soy oil, drained (*Underwood*), 3 oz. 220
in soya oil, drained (*King Oscar*), about 3 pieces 120
in tomato sauce (*Goya*), ¼ cup 130
in tomato sauce (*Underwood*), 3¾ oz. 180
Sauce, see specific listings
Sauerkraut, canned:
(*Boar's Head*), 2 tbsp. 5
(*Claussen*), ¼ cup 5
(*Rosoff* Home Style), ½ cup 50
(*Seneca*), 2 tbsp. 5
Bavarian style (*Seneca*), 2 tbsp. 10
Sauerkraut juice (*Stokely*), 8 fl. oz. 20
Sausage (see also specific listings), cooked:
(*Hormel Special Recipe*), 1 link 111
beef (*Jones Dairy Farm* Golden Brown), 2 links 170
beef, smoked (*Oscar Mayer* Smokies), 1 link 120

brown and serve, beef, smoked (*Jones Dairy Farm*),
  2 links 180
brown and serve, light (*Jones Dairy Farm*), 2 links 110
brown and serve, pork (*Jones Dairy Farm*), 2 links 190
cheese, smoked (*Oscar Mayer* Smokies), 1 link 130
dinner (*Jones Dairy Farm* All Natural), 1 link 130
dinner, Italian (*Jones Dairy Farm*), 1 link 140
patty, sandwich (*Jones Dairy Farm*), 1 patty 140
pork (*Jones Dairy Farm* All Natural Light), 2 links 130
pork, all flavors (*Jones Dairy Farm* Golden Brown),
  2 links 190
pork, light (*Jones Dairy Farm* Golden Brown), 2 links . . 110
pork, patty (*Jones Dairy Farm* All Natural), 1 patty 130
pork, patty (*Jones Dairy Farm* Golden Brown), 1 patty . . 150
smoked (*Oscar Mayer* Smokie Links), 1 link 130
"Sausage," vegetarian, frozen:
(*Green Giant Harvest Burger* Breakfast), 3 links 120
(*Green Giant Harvest Burger* Breakfast), 2 patties 100
Sausage biscuit, frozen, 1 piece:
(*Hormel Quick Meal*) 350
(*Weight Watchers*) 230
w/cheese (*Hormel Quick Meal*) 410
w/egg (*Hormel Quick Meal*) 390
Sausage gravy mix (*Durkee/French's*), ¼ cup* 35
Sausage seasoning (*Tone's*), 1 tsp. 12
Sausage stick, 1 piece
(*Tombstone* Snappy Sticks) 110
beef (*Tombstone* Jerky) 35
beef (*Tombstone* Stick) 110
Scallion, see "Onion, green"
Scallop squash, boiled, drained, sliced, ½ cup 14
Scallops, meat only:
raw, 4 oz. 100
frozen (*Tyson* Delight), ½ cup 80
Scallops, fried, frozen (*Mrs. Paul's*), 12 pieces 200
Scrapple (*Jones Dairy Farm*), 2 oz. 120
Scrod, fresh, see "Cod, Atlantic"
Scup, meat only, 4 oz.:
raw 119
baked, broiled, or microwaved 153

Sea bass, meat only, 4 oz.:

raw 110

baked, broiled, or microwaved 141

Sea trout, meat only, 4 oz.:

raw 118

baked, broiled, or microwaved 151

Seafood, see specific listings

Seafood sauce (see also specific listings), cocktail:

(*Crosse & Blackwell*), ¼ cup 110

(*Del Monte*), ¼ cup 100

(*Heinz*), ¼ cup 60

(*Nalley*), ¼ cup 65

(*Sauceworks*), ¼ cup 60

Seasoning/coating mix (see also specific listings):

country (*Shake 'n Bake*), ⅛ pkt. 35

glaze, honey, tangy or mustard (*Shake 'n Bake*), ⅛ pkt. . . 45

Italian herb (*Shake 'n Bake*), ⅛ pkt. 40

Seaweed:

agar, flakes or bar (*Eden*), 1 tbsp. 10

kombu (*Eden*), ½ of 7″ piece 10

nori (*Eden*), 1 sheet 10

wakame (*Eden/Eden* Flakes), ½ cup 25

Seitan mix (*Arrowhead Mills*), ⅓ cup 150

Semolina flour, mix (*Arrowhead Mills*), ½ cup 240

Sesame butter (*Roaster Fresh*), 1 oz. 168

Sesame paste (see also "Tahini"), whole seed, 1 tbsp. . . 95

Sesame seasoning, all varieties (*Eden*), ½ tsp. 10

Sesame seeds, raw (*McCormick*), ¼ tsp. 2

Shad, American, meat only, 4 oz.:

raw 223

baked, broiled, or microwaved 286

Shallot:

fresh or stored, peeled, chopped, 1 tbsp. 7

freeze-dried (*McCormick*), ¼ tsp. 3

Shark, meat only, raw, 4 oz. 148

Sheepshead, meat only, 4 oz.:

raw 123

baked, broiled, or microwaved 143

Shells, pasta, mix, white cheddar (*Pasta Roni*), approx.

1 cup* 390

Shells, pasta, stuffed, w/out sauce, frozen:
(*Celentano*), 4 shells 330
(*Celentano* Value Pack), 3 shells 240
Shells, pasta, stuffed, dinner, marinara, frozen (*Healthy
   Choice*), 12 oz. 380
Shells, pasta, stuffed, entree, frozen:
(*Celentano*), 10-oz. pkg. 400
(*Celentano* Great Choice), 10-oz. pkg. 250
broccoli (*Celentano* Great Choice), 10-oz. pkg. 190
cheese (*Lean Cuisine* 80 oz.), 8.9-oz. pkg. 210
Florentine (*Celentano*), 10-oz. pkg. 240
Sherbet (see also "Ice" and "Sorbet"), ½ cup:
all flavors (*Breyers*) 120
orange (*Sealtest* Cup) 130
Sherbet pop, 1 piece:
orange (*Popsicle Pop Ups*) 80
rainbow (*Popsicle Pop Ups*) 90
smoothie, strawberry fields (*Dreyer's*) 100
smoothie, tropical oasis (*Dreyer's*) 90
Shortening, 1 tbsp.:
(*Pillsbury Jewel/Snowdrift/Swiftening*) 110
vegetable, regular or butter flavor (*Crisco*) 110
Shrimp, meat only:
fresh, raw, 4 oz. 120
fresh, boiled or steamed, 4 oz. 112
canned, all sizes (*Goya*), 2 oz. 44
frozen, cooked, regular or tail on (*Contessa*), 3 oz. 60
"Shrimp," imitation, frozen, jumbo (*Captain Jac Shrimp
   Tasties*), 3 pieces, 3 oz. 90
Shrimp chow mein, canned (*La Choy* Bi-Pack),1 cup 55
Shrimp cocktail (*Sau-Sea*), 4-oz. jar 100
Shrimp dinner, frozen:
marinara (*Healthy Choice*), 10.5-oz. pkg. 220
Mariner (*The Budget Gourmet*), 11-oz. pkg. 270
vegetables Maria (*Healthy Choice*), 12.5-oz. pkg. 270
Shrimp entree, frozen:
batter, beer (*Gorton's*), 6 pieces 250
breaded (*Mrs. Paul's*), 1 pkg. 350
breaded (*Van de Kamp's*), 7 pieces, 4 oz. 240
breaded, butterfly (*Van de Kamp's*), 7 pieces 280

Shrimp entree, frozen *(cont.)*

breaded, w/pasta (*Marie Callender's*), 1 cup, 7.5 oz.	300
marinara (*Smart Ones*), 9 oz.	190
popcorn, breaded (*Van de Kamp's*), 20 pieces, 4 oz.	270
Shrimp entree mix, Creole (*Luzianne*), 1/5 pkg.	150
Shrimp sauce (*Crosse & Blackwell*), 1/4 cup	110
Shrimp spice (*Tone's* Craboil), 1 tsp.	10

Sizzler, 1 serving:

hot entrees:

chicken breast, hibachi, w/pineapple, 5 oz.	193
chicken breast, lemon-herb, 5 oz.	140
chicken breast, Santa Fe, 5 oz.	150
chicken patty, Malibu	310
hamburger on bun, w/lettuce, tomato	626
salmon, 8 oz.	247
shrimp, broiled, 5 oz.	150
shrimp, fried, 4 pieces	223
shrimp, mini, 4 oz.	152
shrimp scampi, 5 oz.	143
steak, Dakota Ranch, 6 oz.	316
steak, Dakota Ranch, 8 oz.	421
steak, Dakota Ranch, 9.5 oz.	500
swordfish, 8 oz.	315

side dishes:

cheese toast	273
french fries, 4 oz.	358
potato, baked, pulp	105
rice pilaf, 6 oz.	256

sauces, 1 1/2 oz.:

buttery dipping sauce	330
cocktail sauce	40
hibachi sauce	57
Malibu sauce	283
sour dressing	89
tartar sauce	170

hot bar:

chicken wings, 1 oz.	73
focaccia, 2 pieces	108
marinara sauce, 1 oz.	13
meatballs, 4 pieces	157

nacho sauce, 2 oz. 120
pasta, fettuccine, 2 oz. 80
pasta, spaghetti, 2 oz. 80
potato skins, 2 oz. 160
refried beans, ¼ cup 62
saltines, 2 pieces 25
taco filling, 2 oz. 103
taco shells, 1 piece 50
hot bar, soup, 4 oz.:
broccoli cheese 139
chicken noodle soup 31
clam chowder 118
minestrone soup 36
vegetable sirloin 60
salads, prepared, 2 oz.:
carrot and raisin 130
Chinese chicken 54
jicama, spicy 16
Mediterranean Minted Fruit 29
Mexican Fiesta 54
potato, old-fashioned 84
potato, red herb 121
pasta, seafood Louis 64
seafood Louis 56
teriyaki beef 49
tuna pasta 133
dressings, 1 oz.:
blue cheese 111
guacamole 42
honey mustard 160
Italian, lite 14
Parmesan, Italian 100
ranch 120
ranch, lite 90
rice vinegar, Japanese 10
salsa 7
sour dressing 60
Thousand Island 143
Smelt, rainbow, meat only, 4 oz.:
raw 110

Smelt *(cont.)*

baked, broiled, or microwaved 141

Snack bar (see also "Granola and cereal bar"), 1 bar:

(*Little Debbie Star Crunch*) 280

blueberry (*Little Debbie Fruit Boosters*) 190

blueberry (*Sweet Rewards*) 120

brownie (*Sweet Rewards*) 100

brownie, chocolate chip, chocolate raspberry, or peanut

    butter (*Sweet Success Chewy*) 120

fig (*Little Debbie Figaroos*) 180

fudge, double (*Sweet Rewards*) 100

raspberry or strawberry (*Sweet Rewards*) 120

strawberry (*Little Debbie Fruit Boosters*) 190

Snack chips and crisps (see also specific listings):

(*Zings* Chips), 1.8-oz. bag 240

apple cinnamon (*Crunchwells Crumpet Chips*), 1 oz. . . . 110

hot and spicy (*Eden* Wasabi), 1.1 oz. 130

mixed (*Terra* Chips), 1 oz. 140

onion (*Funyons*), 1 oz. 140

Parmesan garlic (*Crunchwells Crumpet Chips*), 1 oz. . . . 100

raspberry (*Crunchwells Crumpet Chips*), 1 oz. 110

spicy barbecue (*Crunchwells Crumpet Chips*), 1 oz. 100

Snack mix:

(*Cheez-It*), ½ cup 140

(*Chex Mix*), ⅔ cup 130

(*Chex Mix* Bold n' Zesty), ½ cup 150

cheddar (*Chex Mix*), ⅔ cup 140

Snail, sea, see "Whelk"

Snapper, meat only, 4 oz.:

raw 113

baked, broiled, or microwaved 145

Snow pea, see "Peas, edible-podded"

Snow pea sprouts (*Jonathan's*), 1 cup 40

Soft drinks, carbonated, 12 fl. oz., except as noted:

apple (*Welch's* Sparkling) 200

birch beer (*Canada Dry*), 8 fl. oz. 110

(*Canada Dry* Hi-Spot/Cactus Cooler), 8 fl. oz. 110

cherry (*Crush*) 200

cherry (*Sunkist*), 8 fl. oz. 140

cherry, black (*Canada Dry*), 8 fl. oz. 130

cherry, black (*Shasta*) 170
cherry, spice (*Slice*) 150
cherry, wild (*Canada Dry*), 8 fl. oz. 110
cherry-lime (*Slice*) 160
chocolate (*Yoo-Hoo*), 9 fl. oz. 150
citrus (*Sunkist*), 8 fl. oz. 100
club soda (*Shasta*) 0
cola (*Canada Dry* Jamaica), 8 fl. oz. 110
cola (*Coca-Cola* Classic), 8 fl. oz. 100
cola (*Pepsi/Pepsi* Caffeine Free) 150
cola (*Shasta*) 170
cola (*Slice*) 160
cola, cherry, wild (*Pepsi*) 160
collins mixer (*Canada Dry/Schweppes*), 8 fl. oz. 100
cranberry (*Shasta*) 180
cream (*Mug*) 170
cream (*Shasta*) 190
cream, vanilla (*Crush*) 180
(*Dr Pepper*) 160
(*Dr. Slice*) 140
fruit punch (*Canada Dry* Tahitian), 8 fl. oz. 150
fruit punch (*Slice*) 190
fruit punch (*Sunkist*), 8 fl. oz. 130
fruit punch, tropical (*Spree*) 170
ginger ale (*Canada Dry/Schweppes*), 8 fl. oz. 90
ginger ale (*Canada Dry* Cherry/Golden), 8 fl. oz. 100
ginger ale, cranberry or lemon (*Canada Dry*), 8 fl. oz. . . 90
ginger ale, grape or raspberry (*Schweppes*), 8 fl. oz. . . . 100
ginger beer (*Schweppes*), 8 fl. oz. 100
grape (*Crush*) 200
grape (*Schweppes*), 8 fl. oz. 130
grape (*Slice*) 190
grape (*Weich's* Sparkling) 200
grapefruit (*Spree*) 170
grapefruit (*Wink*), 8 fl. oz. 130
kiwi-strawberry (*Shasta*) 170
lemon, bitter or sour (*Schweppes*), 8 fl. oz. 110
lemon, sour (*Canada Dry*), 8 fl. oz. 100
lemon-lime (*Slice*) 150
lemon-lime (*Spree*) 170

Soft drinks *(cont.)*

lime (*Canada Dry* Island), 8 fl. oz. 140
lime-lemon (*Shasta Twist*) 150
mandarin-lime (*Spree*) 170
(*Mountain Dew/Mountain Dew* Caffeine Free) 170
orange (*Crush*) 200
orange (*Orangina*), 10 fl. oz. 120
orange (*Sunkist*), 8 fl. oz. 140
orange (*Welch's* Sparkling) 200
orange, mandarin (*Slice*) 190
peach (*Shasta*) 170
peach (*Sunkist*), 8 fl. oz. 120
peach (*Welch's* Sparkling) 220
pineapple (*Crush*) 200
pineapple (*Slice*) 190
pineapple (*Welch's* Sparkling) 210
pineapple-orange (*Shasta*) 180
raspberry creme (*Shasta*) 170
red (*Slice*) 190
root beer (*A&W*), 8 fl. oz. 110
root beer (*Hires*) 180
root beer (*Mug*) 160
seltzer, all flavors (*Canada Dry/Schweppes*) 0
(*7Up/7Up* Cherry) 160
sour mixer (*Canada Dry*), 8 fl. oz. 90
strawberry (*Crush*) 180
strawberry (*Shasta*) 190
strawberry (*Slice*) 170
strawberry (*Welch's* Sparkling) 200
(*Surge*) 170
tonic, all flavors (*Schweppes*), 8 fl. oz. 90
tonic, plain or w/lime (*Canada Dry*), 8 fl. oz. 100
Sole:
fresh, see "Flatfish"
frozen (*Van de Kamp's* Natural), 4-oz. fillet 110
frozen, breaded (*Mrs. Paul's* Premium), 2.9-oz. fillet . . . 170
Sole entree, breaded, frozen, 1 fillet:
(*Mrs. Paul's* Premium) 250
(*Van de Kamp's* Light) 220
Sopressata (*Boar's Head Cinghiale* Mini), 1 oz. 100

Sorbet (see also "Ice" and "Sherbet"), ½ cup:
banana strawberry (*Häagen-Dazs*) 140
cherry cordial (*Edy's/Dreyer's* Whole Fruit) 160
chocolate (*Häagen-Dazs*) 130
cranberry orange (*Ben & Jerry's*) 130
and cream, orange or raspberry (*Häagen-Dazs*) 190
devil's food (*Ben & Jerry's*) 160
lemon (*Edy's/Dreyer's* Whole Fruit) 140
lemon (*Häagen-Dazs Zesty Lemon*) 120
mango (*Häagen-Dazs*) 120
mango lime (*Ben & Jerry's*) 130
mango orange (*Edy's/Dreyer's* Whole Fruit) 120
passion fruit, purple (*Ben & Jerry's*) 120
peach (*Edy's/Dreyer's* Whole Fruit) 130
peach (*Häagen-Dazs* Orchard) 140
piña colada (*Ben & Jerry's*) 140
raspberry (*Edy's/Dreyer's* Whole Fruit) 130
raspberry (*Häagen-Dazs*) 120
strawberry (*Edy's/Dreyer's* Whole Fruit) 120
strawberry (*Häagen-Dazs*) 130
strawberry kiwi (*Ben & Jerry's*) 130
Sorbet bar, 1 bar:
chocolate (*Häagen-Dazs*) 80
wild berry (*Häagen-Dazs*) 90
Sorbet-yogurt bar, 1 bar:
banana and strawberry (*Häagen-Dazs*) 90
chocolate and cherry (*Häagen-Dazs*) 100
raspberry and vanilla (*Häagen-Dazs*) 90
Sorghum syrup, 1 tbsp. 61
Sorrel, see "Dock"
Soup, canned, ready-to-serve, 1 cup, except as noted:
bean, black (*Goya*) 210
bean, black (*Progresso*) 170
bean, black, w/bacon (*Old El Paso*) 160
bean, salsa (*Campbell's* Home Cookin') 160
bean w/bacon (*Campbell's* Microwave), 10½ oz. 280
bean and ham (*Campbell's* Chunky) 190
bean and ham (*Progresso*) 160
beef, barley (*Progresso*) 130
beef, hearty (*Old El Paso*) 120

Soup, canned, ready-to-serve *(cont.)*

beef, minestrone or noodle (*Progresso*) 140
beef, pasta (*Campbell's* Chunky) 150
beef broth (*College Inn*) 20
beef chowder, chunky (*Nalley*), 7½-oz. can 110
beef Stroganoff (*Campbell's* Chunky), 10¾ oz. 310
beef vegetable (*Progresso* 99% Fat Free) 160
beef vegetable country (*Campbell's* Chunky) 160
beef vegetable and rotini (*Progresso*) 130
borscht (*Gold's*) 70
broccoli and shells (*Progresso* Pasta Soup) 80
cheddar potato, white (*Progresso* 99% Fat Free) 140
chicken (*Progresso* Chickarina) 120
chicken, barley or minestrone (*Progresso*) 100
chicken, broccoli cheese (*Campbell's* Chunky) 200
chicken, cream of (*Campbell's* Home Cookin') 210
chicken, rotisserie, seasoned (*Progresso*) 100
chicken, w/vegetables, hearty (*Campbell's* Chunky) . . . 90
chicken, w/vegetables, homestyle (*Progresso*) 80
chicken broth (*College Inn/College Inn* Less Sodium) . . . 25
chicken broth (*Swanson*) 30
chicken chowder (*Nalley*), 7½ oz. 120
chicken chowder, corn (*Campbell's Healthy Request*) . . . 140
chicken chowder, mushroom (*Campbell's* Chunky) 210
chicken noodle (*Campbell's* Chunky Classic) 130
chicken noodle (*Campbell's* Home Cookin') 100
chicken noodle (*Progresso*) 80
chicken noodle (*Progresso* 99% Fat Free) 90
chicken noodle (*Weight Watchers*), 10½ oz. 150
chicken noodle, chunky (*Campbell's* Microwave),
    1 cont. 160
chicken noodle, hearty (*Campbell's Healthy Request*) . . . 160
chicken noodle, hearty (*Old El Paso*) 110
chicken pasta (*Campbell's* Glass Jar) 90
chicken pasta, w/mushroom (*Campbell's* Chunky) 120
chicken and penne, spicy (*Progresso* Pasta Soup) 110
chicken rice (*Campbell's* Chunky) 140
chicken rice (*Campbell's* Home Cookin') 110
chicken rice (*Campbell's* Microwave), 10¾ oz. 120
chicken rice (*Campbell's Healthy Request*) 100

chicken rice (*Old El Paso*) 90
chicken rice (*Weight Watchers*), 10½ oz. 110
chicken rice, w/vegetables (*Progresso*) 100
chicken rice, w/vegetables (*Progresso* 99% Fat Free) 90
chicken rice, wild rice (*Progresso*) 90
chicken rice, chicken and rotini (*Progresso* Pasta Soup) . .90
chicken vegetable (*Campbell's* Chunky) 130
chicken vegetable (*Campbell's* Home Cookin') 130
chicken vegetable (*Old El Paso*) 110
chicken vegetable (*Progresso*) 100
chicken vegetable, hearty (*Campbell's Healthy
  Request*) 120
chicken vegetable, spicy (*Campbell's* Chunky) 90
chili beef w/beans (*Campbell's* Chunky), 11 oz. 300
clam chowder, Manhattan (*Bookbinder's*), ½ cup 80
clam chowder, Manhattan (*Campbell's* Chunky) 130
clam chowder, Manhattan (*Progresso*) 110
clam chowder, New England (*Bookbinder's*), ½ cup . . . 120
clam chowder, New England (*Campbell's* Chunky) 240
clam chowder, New England (*Campbell's* Home
  Cookin') 200
clam chowder, New England (*Campbell's Healthy
  Request*) 120
clam chowder, New England (*Nalley*), 7½ oz. 140
clam chowder, New England (*Progresso*) 200
clam chowder, New England (*Progresso* 99% Fat
  Free) 130
clam and rotini chowder (*Progresso* Pasta Soup) 190
crab bisque (*Bookbinder's*), ½ cup 120
egg flower (*Rice Road*) 90
escarole, in chicken broth (*Progresso*) 25
hot and sour (*Rice Road*) 90
lentil (*Progresso*) 140
lentil (*Progresso* 99% Fat Free) 130
lentil, savory (*Campbell's* Home Cookin') 130
lentil and shells (*Progresso* Pasta Soup) 130
lobster bisque (*Bookbinder's*), ½ cup 90
macaroni and bean (*Progresso*) 160
meatballs and pasta pearls (*Progresso*) 140
minestrone (*Campbell's* Chunky) 140

Soup, canned, ready-to-serve *(cont.)*

minestrone (*Campbell's* Glass Jar/Home Cookin') 120
minestrone (*Progresso*) 120
minestrone (*Progresso* 99% Fat Free) 130
minestrone (*Weight Watchers*), 10½ oz. 130
minestrone, hearty (*Campbell's Healthy Request*) 120
minestrone, Parmesan (*Progresso*) 100
minestrone, Tuscany (*Campbell's* Home Cookin') 160
mushroom, cream of (*Campbell's* Glass Jar) 260
mushroom, cream of (*Campbell's* Home Cookin') 170
mushroom, cream of (*Progresso*) 130
mushroom chicken, creamy (*Progresso* 99% Fat Free) . . 90
mushroom rice (*Campbell's* Home Cookin') 80
oyster stew (*Bookbinder's*), ½ can 90
pasta, Chinese (*Rice Road*) 70
pea, split (*Progresso* 99% Fat Free) 170
pea, split, green (*Progresso*) 170
pea, split, w/ham (*Campbell's* Chunky) 190
pea, split, w/ham (*Campbell's* Home Cookin') 170
pea, split, w/ham (*Campbell's Healthy Request*) 170
pea, split, w/ham (*Progresso*) 150
penne, hearty, in chicken broth (*Progresso* Pasta
  Soup) 90
penne, zesty (*Campbell's Healthy Request*) 90
pepper steak (*Campbell's* Chunky) 140
potato, w/roasted garlic (*Campbell's* Home Cookin') 180
potato ham chowder (*Campbell's*) 220
potato ham chowder (*Campbell's* Chunky), 10¾ oz. . . . 270
seafood bisque (*Bookbinder's*), ½ cup 140
shrimp bisque (*Bookbinder's*), ½ cup 120
sirloin burger, w/vegetable (*Campbell's* Chunky) 190
snapper (*Bookbinder's*), ½ cup 110
steak and potato (*Campbell's* Chunky) 160
tomato, garden (*Campbell's* Home Cookin'), 10¾ oz. . . . 150
tomato, hearty, and rotini (*Progresso* Pasta Soup) 130
tomato, tortellini (*Progresso* Pasta Soup) 120
tomato, vegetable (*Campbell's* Glass Jar) 80
tomato, vegetable (*Progresso*) 90
tomato, vegetable, garden (*Progresso* 99% Fat Free) . . . 100

tomato, vegetable, w/pasta (*Campbell's Healthy Request*) 120
tortellini, in chicken broth (*Progresso*) 70
tortellini, w/chicken and vegetables (*Campbell's*) 110
turkey w/wild rice (*Campbell's Healthy Request*) 120
vegetable (*Campbell's* Chunky) 130
vegetable (*Progresso*) 90
vegetable (*Progresso* 99% Fat Free) 80
vegetable (*Weight Watchers*), 10½ oz. 130
vegetable, country (*Campbell's* Home Cookin') 110
vegetable, garden (*Old El Paso*) 110
vegetable, harborside (*Campbell's* Home Cookin') 80
vegetable, hearty (*Campbell's Healthy Request*) 100
vegetable, hearty, w/pasta (*Campbell's* Chunky) 130
vegetable, hearty, w/rotini (*Progresso* Pasta Soup) 110
vegetable, Italian (*Campbell's* Home Cookin') 100
vegetable, and pasta (*Campbell's* Glass Jar) 110
vegetable, Southwestern (*Campbell's* Home Cookin') ... 130
vegetable, Southwestern, w/black bean (*Campbell's Healthy Request*) 140
vegetable beef (*Campbell's* Chunky) 150
vegetable beef (*Campbell's* Home Cookin') 120
vegetable beef (*Campbell's* Low Sodium), 10¾ oz. 160
vegetable beef (*Campbell's* Microwave), 1 cont. 140
vegetable beef, hearty (*Campbell's Healthy Request*) ... 140
vegetable broth (*Swanson*) 20
Soup, canned, condensed, undiluted, ½ cup:
asparagus, cream of (*Campbell's*) 90
bean, black (*Campbell's*) 120
bean w/bacon (*Campbell's*) 180
bean w/bacon (*Campbell's Healthy Request*) 150
beef broth, double rich (*Campbell's*) 15
beef consommé (*Campbell's*) 25
beef noodle (*Campbell's*) 70
beef w/vegetables and barley (*Campbell's*) 80
broccoli, cream of (*Campbell's*) 100
broccoli, cream of (*Campbell's* 98% Fat Free) 80
broccoli, cream of (*Campbell's Healthy Request*) 70
broccoli, creamy (*Campbell's Healthy Request Creative Chef*) 70

Soup, canned, condensed *(cont.)*

broccoli cheese (*Campbell's*) 110
celery, cream of (*Campbell's*) 110
celery, cream of (*Campbell's 98% Fat Free*) 70
celery, cream of (*Campbell's Healthy Request*) 70
cheese (*Campbell's 98% Fat Free*) 80
cheese, cheddar (*Campbell's*) 90
cheese, nacho (*Campbell's*) 140
chicken, cream of:
  (*Campbell's*) 130
  (*Campbell's 98% Fat Free*) 80
  (*Campbell's Healthy Request*) 70
  (*Campbell's Healthy Request Creative Chef*) 80
  and broccoli (*Campbell's*) 120
  and broccoli (*Campbell's Healthy Request*) 80
chicken alphabet, w/vegetables (*Campbell's*) 80
chicken broth (*Campbell's*) 30
chicken and dumplings (*Campbell's*) 80
chicken gumbo (*Campbell's*) 60
chicken mushroom, creamy (*Campbell's*) 130
chicken noodle (*Campbell's/Campbell's Healthy
Request*) 70
chicken noodle, creamy (*Campbell's*) 130
chicken noodle, curly or noodle O's (*Campbell's*) 80
chicken noodle, homestyle (*Campbell's*) 70
chicken w/rice (*Campbell's*) 70
chicken w/rice (*Campbell's Healthy Request*) 60
chicken and stars (*Campbell's*) 70
chicken vegetable (*Campbell's/Campbell's Healthy
Request*) 80
chicken vegetable, Southwestern (*Campbell's*) 110
chicken wild rice (*Campbell's*) 70
chili beef w/beans (*Campbell's*) 170
clam chowder, Manhattan (*Campbell's*) 60
clam chowder, New England (*Campbell's*) 100
clam chowder, New England (*Doxsee*) 90
corn, golden (*Campbell's*) 120
minestrone (*Campbell's*) 100
minestrone (*Campbell's Healthy Request*) 90
mushroom, beefy (*Campbell's*) 70

mushroom, cream of (*Campbell's*) 110
mushroom, cream of (*Campbell's 98% Fat Free*) 70
mushroom, cream of (*Campbell's Healthy Request*) 70
mushroom, cream of (*Campbell's Healthy Request
    Creative Chef*) 70
mushroom, golden (*Campbell's*) 80
noodle, curly, chicken broth (*Campbell's*) 80
noodle, double, chicken broth (*Campbell's*) 100
noodle and ground beef (*Campbell's*) 100
onion, creamy (*Campbell's*) 110
onion, French, w/beef stock (*Campbell's*) 70
oyster stew (*Campbell's*) 90
pea, green, or split pea w/ham and bacon
    (*Campbell's*) 180
pepper, cream of Mexican (*Campbell's*) 110
pepperpot (*Campbell's*) 100
potato, cream of (*Campbell's*) 90
potato, cream of (*Campbell's Healthy Request Creative
    Chef*) 80
Scotch broth (*Campbell's*) 80
shrimp, cream of (*Campbell's*) 100
tomato (*Campbell's*) 100
tomato (*Campbell's Healthy Request*) 90
tomato, cream of (*Campbell's* Homestyle) 110
tomato, fiesta (*Campbell's*) 70
tomato, Italian, w/basil, oregano (*Campbell's*) 100
tomato bisque (*Campbell's*) 130
tomato w/herbs (*Campbell's Healthy Request Creative
    Chef*) 100
tomato rice (*Campbell's* Old Fashioned) 120
turkey, noodle or vegetable (*Campbell's*) 80
vegetable (*Campbell's* 10¾ oz.) 80
vegetable (*Campbell's Healthy Request*) 90
vegetable (*Campbell's* Old Fashioned) 70
vegetable, California style (*Campbell's*) 60
vegetable, hearty (*Campbell's Healthy Request*) 90
vegetable, hearty, w/pasta (*Campbell's*) 90
vegetable, vegetarian (*Campbell's*) 70
vegetable beef (*Campbell's/Campbell's Healthy Request*) . . 80
won ton (*Campbell's*) 45

Soup, frozen, 7.5 oz., except as noted:
barley mushroom (*Tabatchnick/Tabatchnick* No Salt) 70
bean, Yankee (*Tabatchnick*) 160
broccoli, cream of (*Tabatchnick*) 90
cabbage (*Tabatchnick*) 60
cheddar vegetable, Wisconsin (*Tabatchnick*) 140
cheese, Wisconsin (*Schwan's*), 1 cup 210
chicken w/noodles and dumplings (*Tabatchnick*) 70
chicken w/noodles and vegetables (*Tabatchnick*) 35
clam chowder, Boston (*Schwan's*), 1 cup 180
corn chowder or minestrone (*Tabatchnick*) 150
lentil, Tuscany (*Tabatchnick*) 140
pea (*Tabatchnick/Tabatchnick* No Salt) 180
potato, New England (*Tabatchnick*) 150
potato, old-fashioned (*Tabatchnick*) 70
spinach, cream of (*Tabatchnick*) 90
vegetable or vegetable, no salt (*Tabatchnick*) 110
Soup mix, dry, 1 pkg. or cont., except as noted:
barley, beef (*Buckeye Beans*), 1 cup* 170
bean (*Buckeye Beans*), 1 cup* 170
bean, black (*Knorr* Cup) 190
bean, black, hearty (*Fantastic* Cup) 210
bean, navy (*Knorr* Cup) 130
bean, vegetable (*Buckeye Beans*), 1 cup* 150
beef vegetable (*Hamburger Helper*), 1 cup* 190
broccoli, cream of (*Knorr* Chef's), 2 tbsp. 60
broccoli-cheddar, creamy (*Fantastic* Cup) 130
broccoli-cheese, creamy (*Cup-a-Soup*) 70
chicken, cream of (*Cup-a-Soup*) 70
chicken, hearty, supreme (*Cup-a-Soup*) 90
chicken, onion and rice (*Kettle Creations*), ¼ pkg. 120
chicken, pasta and beans (*Kettle Creations*), ¼ pkg. . . . 110
chicken, thyme (*Buckeye Beans*), 1 cup* 180
chicken noodle (*Campbell's* Real Chicken Broth),
   3 tbsp. 100
chicken noodle (*Campbell's* Soup and Recipe), 3 tbsp. . . . 90
chicken noodle (*Cup-a-Soup*) 50
chicken noodle, double (*Campbell's*) 170
chicken noodle, hearty (*Cup-a-Soup*) 60
chili, black bean (*Buckeye Beans*), 1 cup* 180

chili, chicken, white (*Buckeye Beans*), 1 cup* 290
chili, hearty (*Fantastic Cha-Cha* Cup) 220
chili, vegetarian (*Fantastic*), ½ cup* 50
clam chowder, New England (*Knorr* Chef's), 3 tbsp. 90
corn chowder (*Knorr* Cup) 140
corn potato chowder, creamy (*Fantastic* Cup) 170
couscous (*Casbah* Moroccan Stew Cup) 180
couscous, black bean salsa (*Fantastic* Cup) 240
couscous, cheddar, nacho (*Fantastic* Cup) 200
couscous, corn, sweet (*Fantastic* Cup) 180
couscous, w/lentils (*Fantastic* Only A Pinch Cup) 220
couscous, w/lentils, hearty (*Fantastic*) 230
couscous, vegetable, Creole (*Fantastic* Cup) 220
herb, fine (*Knorr* Box), 2 tbsp. 100
hot and sour (*Knorr* Box), 2 tbsp. 45
leek (*Knorr* Box), 2 tbsp. 70
lentil, hearty (*Fantastic*), ⅔ oz. 230
lentil, hearty (*Knorr* Cup) 220
minestrone (*Kettle Creations*), ¼ pkg. 110
minestrone, hearty (*Fantastic* Cup) 150
minestrone, hearty (*Knorr* Cup) 120
mushroom, cream of (*Cup-a-Soup*) 60
mushroom, creamy (*Fantastic* Cup) 120
noodle, chicken free (*Fantastic* Cup) 140
noodle, homestyle (*Borden*), ¼ pkg. 70
noodle, rings (*Cup-a-Soup*) 50
noodle, beef (*Campbell's* Baked Ramen) 210
noodle, beef (*Campbell's/Sanwa* Ramen), ½ block 170
noodle, chicken (*Campbell's* Baked Ramen) 210
noodle, chicken (*Knorr* Box), 2 tbsp. 90
noodle, chicken (*Knorr* Cup) 110
noodle, chicken (*Sanwa* Ramen Pride), ½ block 170
noodle, chicken, regular or spicy (*Campbell's* Baked
    Ramen), ½ block 140
noodle, chicken, spicy (*Campbell's* Ramen), ½ block . . . 170
noodle, Oriental (*Campbell's/Sanwa* Ramen), ½ block . . 170
noodle, pork (*Campbell's* Ramen), ½ block 170
noodle, shrimp (*Campbell's/Sanwa* Ramen), ½ block . . . 170
noodle, vegetable, curry (*Fantastic* Cup) 140
noodle, vegetable, miso (*Fantastic* Cup) 130

Soup mix *(cont.)*

onion (*Campbell's* Soup and Recipe), 1 tbsp. 20
onion (*Knorr* Box), 2 tbsp. 45
oxtail (*Knorr* Box), 2 tbsp. 60
pasta and bean (*Bean Cuisine* Ultima), 1 serving 117
pasta and bean (*Casbah Pasta Fasul*) 160
pasta and bean (*Kettle Creations*), ¼ pkg. 130
pea, green (*Cup-a-Soup*) 110
pea, snow, cream of (*Knorr* Chef's), 3 tbsp. 70
pea, split (*Bean Cuisine* Thick as Fog), 1 serving 116
pea, split (*Buckeye Beans*), 1 cup* 250
pea, split (*Knorr* Cup) 150
pea, split, hearty (*Fantastic* Cup) 190
potato leek (*Knorr* Cup) 120
rice (*Casbah Thai Yum*) 160
rice and beans (*Casbah* La Fiesta) 170
rice and beans, Cajun (*Casbah* Jambalaya) 128
rice and beans, Cajun (*Fantastic* Cup) 240
rice and beans, Caribbean (*Fantastic* Cup) 230
rice and beans, curry (*Fantastic* Cup) 260
rice and beans, Italian (*Fantastic* Cup) 240
rice and beans, Spanish (*Fantastic* Only A Pinch Cup) . . 210
rice and beans, Szechuan (*Fantastic* Cup) 210
rice and beans, Tex-Mex (*Fantastic* Cup) 270
spinach, cream of (*Knorr* Box), 2 tbsp. 70
tomato (*Cup-a-Soup*) 90
tomato basil (*Knorr* Box), 2 tbsp. 80
tomato rice Parmesano (*Fantastic* Cup) 200
tomato vegetable (*Campbell's Soupsations*) 130
vegetable (*Knorr* Box), 2 tbsp. 30
vegetable, chicken flavor (*Cup-a-Soup*) 50
vegetable, chicken flavor (*Knorr* Cup) 100
vegetable, chicken flavor, creamy (*Cup-a-Soup*) 90
vegetable, spring (*Cup-a-Soup*) 45
vegetable, spring (*Knorr*), 2 tbsp. 25
vegetable barley, hearty (*Fantastic* Cup) 150
Soup base, bottled, 1 tsp.:
(*Goya* Recaito) 3
(*Goya* Sofrito) 5

Soup base, mix, ⅛ pkg., except as noted:

beef, ground, vegetable (*Soup Starter*) 80

beef barley vegetable (*Soup Starter*) 100

beef stew, hearty (*Soup Starter*), ⅟₇ pkg. 80

beef vegetable (*Soup Starter*) 90

chicken noodle (*Soup Starter*) 80

chicken and rice (*Soup Starter*) 70

chicken vegetable (*Soup Starter*), ⅟₇ pkg. 70

chicken w/white and wild rice (*Soup Starter*) 70

Sour cream, see "Cream, sour"

Sour cream dip mix (*Durkee*), 2 tsp. 25

Soursop, ½ cup 75

Soy beverage, 8 fl. oz.:

(*EdenSoy/EdenSoy* Extra) 130

(*Soy Moo* Fat Free) 110

carob (*EdenSoy*) 150

vanilla (*EdenSoy/EdenSoy* Extra) 150

Soy beverage mix (*Loma Linda Soyagen*), ¼ cup 130

Soy butter mix (*Morningstar Farms/Natural Touch*

SoyButter), 2 tbsp. 170

Soy flour (*Arrowhead Mills*), ½ cup 200

Soy sauce, 1 tbsp.

(*La Choy*) 10

(*La Choy* Lite) 15

Soybeans:

dried, raw (*Arrowhead Mills*), ¼ cup 170

canned, black (*Eden* Organic), ½ cup 90

Soybean kernels, roasted, toasted, 1 oz. or 95

kernels. 129

Soybean sprouts (*Jonathan's*), 1 cup, 3 oz. 100

Spaghetti, plain, see "Pasta"

Spaghetti dishes, mix:

w/meat sauce (*Kraft* Dinner), 5.5 oz. 330

mild or tangy (*Kraft* American Dinner), 2 oz. 200

Spaghetti entree, canned:

w/franks (*Van Camp's Weenee*), 1 can 230

w/meatballs (*Hormel* Micro Cup), 7½ oz. 210

w/meatballs (*Libby's Diner*), 7¾ oz. 190

w/meatballs (*Top Shelf*), 10 oz. 300

Spaghetti entree, frozen:
marinara (*The Budget Gourmet*), 9 oz. 320
marinara (*Weight Watchers*), 9 oz. 280
meat sauce (*The Budget Gourmet* Special Selections),
   10 oz. 320
meat sauce (*Lean Cuisine*), 11.5 oz. 300
meat sauce (*Stouffer's*), 10 oz. 350
meat sauce (*Weight Watchers*), 10 oz. 290
w/meatballs (*Lean Cuisine*), 9.5 oz. 280
w/meatballs (*Stouffer's*), 12⅝ oz. 440
and sauce, w/seasoned beef (*Healthy Choice*), 10 oz. . . . 260
Spaghetti sauce, see "Pasta sauce"
Spaghetti squash, baked or boiled, drained, ½ cup 23
Spareribs, see "Pork"
Spelt flakes (*Arrowhead Mills*), 1 cup 100
Spinach, ½ cup, except as noted:
fresh, raw, chopped (*Dole*), 1 cup 15
canned (*Del Monte/Del Monte* No Salt) 30
frozen (*Green Giant/Green Giant Harvest Fresh*) 25
frozen, leaf or chopped (*Birds Eye*), ⅓ cup 20
Spinach dishes, frozen:
creamed (*Green Giant*), ½ cup 80
creamed (*Stouffer's* Side Dish), ½ of 9-oz. pkg. 160
soufflé (*Stouffer's* Side Dish), 4 oz. 150
Spinach salad, see "Salad blend mix"
Spiny lobster, meat only, 4 oz.:
raw 127
boiled or steamed 138
Split peas:
boiled, ½ cup 116
green, dry (*Arrowhead Mills*), ¼ cup 170
Sports drink, all flavors:
(*All Sport*), 8 fl. oz. 70
(*Body Works*), 12 fl. oz. 90
Spot, meat only, baked, broiled, or microwaved, 4 oz. . . . 179
Spring onion, see "Onion, green"
Sprouts (see also specific listings):
bean (*Frieda's*), 1 oz. 10
bean, canned (*La Choy*), 1 cup 10
mixed (*Jonathan's* Gourmet), 1 cup, 3 oz. 20

mixed, lentil, adzuki, pea (*Jonathan's*), 3 oz. 100
Squab, fresh, raw, 4 oz.:
meat w/skin 333
breast meat only 161
Squash (see also specific listings):
canned (*Stokely*), ½ cup 50
frozen (*Birds Eye*), ½ cup 50
Squid:
meat only, raw, 4 oz. 104
canned (*Goya*), ⅓ can 45
Steak sauce, 1 tbsp.:
(*A.1.*) 15
(*Alanna* Irish) 15
(*Heinz* Traditional) 10
garlic peppercorn or sweet/spicy (*Lea & Perrins*) 25
New Orleans style (*Trappey's Chef-Magic*) 10
Stir-fry sauce (see also specific listings), 1 tbsp.:
(*House of Tsang* Classic) 25
(*House of Tsang Saigon Sizzle*) 40
(*House of Tsang Szechuan Spicy*) 20
garlic and ginger (*Rice Road*) 25
honey or regular (*Ken's Steak House*) 20
sesame and ginger (*Rice Road*) 15
sweet and sour (*House of Tsang*) 35
teriyaki (*Rice Road*) 20
Stir-fry seasoning, teriyaki flavor (*Adolph's Meal*
  Makers), 1 tbsp. 30
Stomach, pork, raw, 1 oz. 44
Strawberry:
fresh (*Dole*), 8 berries, 5.3 oz. 45
canned, whole, in syrup (*Comstock*), ½ cup 140
frozen (*Birds Eye*), ½ cup 70
Strawberry drink (*Capri Sun* Cooler), 6.75 fl. oz. 100
Strawberry drink blends, 8 fl. oz.:
guava (*Santa Cruz*) 100
melon (*Veryfine* Shivering Chillers) 120
orange banana (*Tree Top*) 120
Strawberry drink mix* (*Kool-Aid*), 8 fl. oz. 100
Strawberry milk beverage:
(*Nestlé Quik*), 8 fl. oz. 230

Strawberry milk beverage *(cont.)*

low-fat (*Nestlé Quik*), 8-fl.-oz. cont. 210

low-fat, banana (*Nestlé Quik*), 8 fl. oz. 200

shake (*Nestlé Killer*), 14 oz. 420

shake (*Nestlé Quik*), 9 oz. 270

Strawberry milk drink mix (*Nestlé Quik*), 2 tbsp. 90

Strawberry nectar:

(*Libby's/Kern's*), 11.5 fl. oz. 210

(*Veryfine* Juice-Ups), 8 fl. oz. 140

banana (*Kern's*), 8 fl. oz. 150

Strawberry pie glaze (*Smucker's*), 2 tbsp. 80

Strawberry syrup (*Hershey's*), 2 tbsp. 100

Strawberry topping (*Mrs. Richardson's* Fat Free),

   2 tbsp. 70

Stroganoff gravy (*Pepperidge Farm*), ¼ cup 30

Stroganoff sauce, beef (*Lawry's*), 1 tbsp. 20

Strudel, apple (*Entenmann's*), ¼ pastry 310

Stuffing (see also "Stuffing mix"):

apple and raisin (*Pepperidge Farm*), ½ cup 140

Cajun rice (*Good Harvest*), ½ cup 130

chicken, classic (*Pepperidge Farm*), ½ cup 130

corn bread (*Pepperidge Farm*), ¾ cup 170

corn bread, honey pecan (*Pepperidge Farm*), ½ cup . . . 140

country style or cube (*Pepperidge Farm*), ¾ cup 140

cube, bread, unseasoned (*Brownberry*), 2 cups 240

garden and herb, country (*Pepperidge Farm*), ½ cup . . . 150

herb seasoned (*Brownberry*), 1 cup 200

herb seasoned (*Pepperidge Farm*), ¾ cup 170

sage and onion (*Brownberry* 7 oz./14 oz.), 2 cups 240

sage and onion (*Pepperidge Farm*), ½ cup 150

Santa Fe or sourdough (*Good Harvest*), ½ cup 110

vegetable, harvest, and almond (*Pepperidge Farm*),

   ½ cup 140

wild rice mushroom (*Pepperidge Farm*), ⅔ cup 170

wild rice trio (*Good Harvest*), ½ cup 140

Stuffing mix, ⅙ box dry, except as noted:

(*Kellogg's Crouettes*), 1 cup 120

all flavors (*Rice-A-Roni*), 1 cup* 170

all flavors (*Stove Top*) 110

chicken flavor (*Stove Top* Microwave) 130

corn bread, homestyle (*Stove Top* Microwave) 120
herb (*Stove Top* Flexible Serve), 1 oz. 120
Sturgeon, meat only, 4 oz.:
raw 120
baked, broiled, or microwaved 153
smoked 196
Succotash, canned, ½ cup:
whole kernel (*S&W*) 100
whole kernel (*Seneca*) 90
Sucker, white, meat only, 4 oz.:
raw 105
baked, broiled, or microwaved 135
Sugar, cane (*Domino*):
brown, light or dark, 1 tsp. 15
powdered, ¼ cup 120
powdered, lemon or strawberry flavored, ¼ cup 110
white, 1 tsp. or 1 pkt. 15
Sugar, maple, 1 oz. 99
Sugar, substitute:
(*Equal*), 1 pkt. 4
(*NutraSweet*), 1 tsp. 2
Sugar snap peas, see "Peas, edible-podded"
Summer sausage:
(*Oscar Mayer*), 2 slices, 1.6 oz. 140
beef (*Oscar Mayer*), 2 slices, 1.6 oz. 140
Summer squash (*Dole*), ½ medium, 3.5 oz. 20
Sunburst squash, raw (*Frieda's*), 1 oz. 4
Sunfish, pumpkinseed, meat only, 4 oz.:
raw 101
baked, broiled, or microwaved 129
Sunflower seed:
(*Frito-Lay*), ⅓ cup 140
dry-roasted, in shell (*Planters* Original), ¾ cup, 1 oz.
   edible 160
dry-roasted, kernels (*Planters*), ¼ cup 190
honey-roasted, kernels (*Planters*), 1.7 oz. 280
oil-roasted or barbecued, kernels (*Planters*), 1.7 oz. . . . 290
Sunflower sprouts (*Jonathan's*), 1 cup 45
Surimi, from walleye pollock, 4 oz. 112
Sweet peas, see "Peas, green"

Sweet potato:

raw (*Dole*), 4.6-oz. potato 130
baked in skin, 1 medium 118
canned (*Seneca* Yams), ½ cup 150
canned, halves (*Royal Prince*), 3 pieces, 5.7 oz. 190
canned, candied (*S&W*), ½ cup 170
canned, candied or orange-pineapple (*Royal Prince*),
  ½ cup 210
frozen (*Mrs. Paul's*), 5 fl. oz. 300
frozen (*Mrs. Paul's* Sweets'n Apples), 1¼ cups 270
Sweet potato chips, plain or cinnamon (*Terra*), 1 oz. . . . 140
Sweet and sour dinner mix (*La Choy*), ¼ pkg. 90
Sweet and sour drink mixer (*Holland House/Mr. & Mrs.
  T/Rose's*), 4 fl. oz. 100
Sweet and sour sauce, 2 tbsp.:
(*Contadina*) 40
(*House of Tsang*) 30
(*Kikkoman*) 35
(*Kraft*) 80
(*La Choy*) 60
(*World Harbors Maui Mountain*) 60
duck sauce (*Ka-Me*) 80
duck sauce (*La Choy*) 60
Sweetbreads, see "Pancreas" and "Thymus"
Swiss chard, ½ cup:
raw, chopped 3
boiled, drained, chopped 18
Swiss steak seasoning mix (*Durkee/French's* Roasting
  Bag), 1/9 pkg. 10
Swordfish, fresh, meat only, 4 oz.:
fresh, raw 137
fresh, baked, broiled, or microwaved 176
frozen, steaks (*Peter Pan*) 160
Syrup, see specific listings
Szechwan sauce (*Ka-Me*), 1 tbsp. 20

T

Taco Bell, tacos and tostadas *(cont.)*

Double Decker Taco Supreme 390
kid's soft taco, chicken 240
kid's soft taco, chicken, light 180
kid's soft taco roll-up 290
soft taco 210
soft taco, chicken 250
soft taco, chicken, light 180
soft taco, steak 200
soft *Taco Supreme* 260
taco 170
Taco Supreme 220
tostada 200
specialty items:
beef *MexiMelt* 300
cinnamon twists 140
Mexican pizza 570
Mexican rice 190
nachos 310
nachos *BellGrande* 750
nachos supreme 430
pintos 'n cheese 190
taco salad 840
taco salad w/out shell 420
sides and condiments:
cheese, cheddar 30
cheese, cheddar, nonfat 10
cheese, pepper jack 25
green sauce or pico de gallo 5
guacamole 35
nacho cheese sauce 120
picante or taco sauce 0
ranch dressing 136
red sauce 10
salsa 25
sour cream 40
sour cream, nonfat 20
Taco John's, 1 serving:
burritos:
bean 387

    beef 449
    combination 418
    meat and potato 503
    ranch 447
    smothered, platter 1,031
    super 465
chimichanga platter 979
enchilada platter, double 967
fajitas, chicken:
    burrito 370
    salad, w/out dressing 557
    soft shell 200
Mexi Rolls w/nacho cheese 863
nachos, super 919
sampler platter 1,406
sierra chicken fillet sandwich 534
tacos:
    crispy 182
    kid's meal, w/crispy taco 579
    kid's meal, w/soft shell taco 617
    soft shell 230
    Taco Bravo 346
    taco burger 280
sides and condiments:
    beans, refried 357
    chili 350
    Mexican rice 567
    nachos 333
    nacho cheese 300
    Potato Oles 363
    Potato Oles, large 484
    Potato Oles, w/nacho cheese 483
    salad dressing, house 114
    sour cream 60
desserts:
    choco taco 320
    churro 147
    flauta, apple 84
    flauta, cherry 143
    flauta, cream cheese 181

Taco John's,* desserts *(cont.)
Italian ice 80
Taco mix, dinner:
(*Old El Paso*), 2 tacos* 270
(*Pancho Villa*), 2 tacos* 270
soft (*Old El Paso*), 2 tacos* 380
Taco sauce:
(*Chi-Chi's* Thick & Chunky), 1 tbsp. 10
(*Pancho Villa*), 2 tbsp. 15
all varieties (*Old El Paso*), 1 tbsp. 5
Taco seasoning (*Tone's*), 2 tsp. 20
Taco seasoning mix:
(*McCormick*), 2 tsp. 20
(*Old El Paso*), 2 tsp. 20
(*Old El Paso* 40% Less Sodium), 2 tsp. 15
(*Pancho Villa*), 2 tsp. 20
salad (*Durkee* Pouch), 1/6 pkg. 20
Taco shell (see also "Tortilla"):
(*Gebhardt*), 3 shells 155
(*Old El Paso* Super), 2 shells 200
(*Pancho Villa*), 3 shells 180
golden or white corn (*Old El Paso*), 3 shells 170
tostada (*Old El Paso*), 3 shells 170
white corn (*Chi-Chi's*), 2 shells 170
Tahini:
(*Arrowhead Mills*), 1 oz. 170
(*Krinos*), 2 tbsp. 260
Tahini sauce mix (*Casbah*), 1 oz. 160
Tamale, canned:
(*Nalley*), 3 pieces 290
(*Van Camp's*), 2 pieces 210
in chili gravy (*Old El Paso*), 3 pieces 320
beef, hot-spicy or regular (*Hormel*), 3 pieces 280
chicken (*Hormel*), 3 pieces 210
Tamale, frozen (*Goya*), 1 piece 300
Tamarind, frozen, chunks (*Goya*), 1/3 pkg. 70
Tamarind nectar, canned (*Goya*), 12 fl. oz. 240
Tangerine:
fresh (*Dole*), 2 fruits 70
canned, in juice (*S&W* Mandarin), 2/3 cup 70

canned, in light syrup (*Dole*), ½ cup 80
Tangerine juice:
blend (*Dole* Mandarin), 8 fl. oz. 140
frozen* (*Minute Maid* Beverage), 8 fl. oz. 120
Tapioca, dry (*Minute*), 1½ tsp. 20
Tapioca pudding, see "Pudding"
Taro, cooked (*Frieda's*), 5 oz. 150
Taro chips, spiced (*Terra*), 1 oz. 130
Tartar sauce, 2 tbsp.:
(*Nalley*) 190
(*Sauceworks*) 100
lemon herb flavor (*Sauceworks*) 150
Tea (see also "Tea, iced"):
plain, regular or instant, all varieties, 1 bag or 1 tsp. 0
flavored, lemon, instant (*Lipton*), 1 tsp. 0
Tea, iced, 8 fl. oz., except as noted:
(*Schweppes*) 90
(*Veryfine* Chillers) 80
all fruit flavors (*Apple & Eve*) 100
lemon (*Tropicana*) 100
peach or raspberry (*Tropicana*), 11.5 fl. oz. 160
peach-kiwi (*Veryfine* Chillers) 80
raspberry (*Veryfine* Chillers) 100
Tea, iced, mix, 1⅔ tbsp.:
lemon flavor (*Lipton*) 90
w/out lemon (*Lipton*) 80
Teff seed or flour (*Arrowhead Mills*), 2 oz. 200
Tempeh, ½ cup 165
Teriyaki entree, frozen (*Lean Cuisine Lunch Classics*),
  10 oz. 270
Teriyaki sauce, 1 tbsp., except as noted:
(*House of Tsang Korean Teriyaki*) 30
(*La Choy/La Choy* Lite/Chun King Hot) 20
(*Rice Road*) 15
cooking, and marinade (*S&W/S&W* Lite) 25
hot (*Mountain Harbors Maui Mountain*), 2 tbsp. 70
marinade and (*Lea & Perrins*) 15
marinade and (*World Harbors Maui Mountain*), 2 tbsp. . . 70
Thai sauce (*World Harbors* Nong Khai), 2 tbsp. 40
Thyme, dried (*McCormick*), ¼ tsp. 4

Thymus, braised, 4 oz.:

beef 362

veal 197

Tilefish, meat only, 4 oz.:

raw 108

baked, broiled, or microwaved 167

Toaster muffins and pastries, 1 piece

apple cinnamon or blueberry (*Pop-Tarts*) 210

apple cinnamon or blueberry (*Thomas' Toast-r-Cakes*) . . 100

banana nut (*Thomas' Toast-r-Cakes*) 110

blueberry or cherry, frosted (*Pop-Tarts*) 200

brown sugar–cinnamon (*Pop-Tarts*) 220

brown sugar–cinnamon, frosted (*Pop-Tarts*) 210

cherry or strawberry (*Pop-Tarts*) 200

chocolate fudge, frosted (*Pop-Tarts*) 200

chocolate-vanilla creme, frosted (*Pop-Tarts*) 200

corn (*Thomas' Toast-r-Cakes*) 110

grape, frosted (*Pop-Tarts*) 200

raisin bran (*Thomas' Toast-r-Cakes*) 90

raspberry, frosted (*Pop-Tarts*) 210

S'mores (*Pop-Tarts*) 200

strawberry (*Thomas' Toast-r-Cakes*) 110

strawberry, frosted (*Pop-Tarts*) 200

Tofu:

fresh, ½ cup 94

fresh, pasteurized (*Frieda's*), 4.2 oz. 86

okara, ½ cup 47

silken (*Nasoya*), ⅕ of 1-lb. block 50

salted and fermented (fuyu), 1 oz. 33

Tofu dishes, mix, dry:

burger (*Fantastic* Classics), ⅛ cup 70

chow mein, Mandarin (*Fantastic* Classics), ⅝ cup 170

shells 'n curry (*Fantastic* Classics), ½ cup 200

Stroganoff, creamy (*Fantastic* Classics), ½ cup 190

Tomatillo, in jars:

(*La Victoria* Entero), 5 pieces 40

crushed (*La Victoria*), 4½ oz. 45

Tomato:

raw (*Dole*), 1 medium, 3.5 oz. 80

raw, chopped, ½ cup 19

boiled, ½ cup 32
dried, see "Tomato, dried"
Tomato, canned, ½ cup, except as noted:
(*Contadina* Pasta Ready) 40
(*Contadina* Recipe Ready) 25
whole (*Del Monte*) 25
whole, Italian pear or peeled (*Contadina*) 25
whole, peeled or w/basil (*Progresso*) 20
aspic (*S&W*) 50
w/cheeses, three (*Contadina* Pasta Ready) 70
chunky, chili (*Del Monte*) 30
chunky, pasta (*Del Monte*) 45
chunky, salsa (*Del Monte*) 35
crushed (*Contadina*), ¼ cup 20
crushed (*Progresso*) 20
diced (*Del Monte/Del Monte* No Salt) 25
diced, w/basil, garlic, oregano (*Del Monte*) 50
diced, w/onion, garlic (*Del Monte*) 35
w/green chilies, diced (*Chi-Chi's*), ¼ cup 20
w/green chilies or jalapeños (*Old El Paso*), ¼ cup 10
w/mushrooms or primavera (*Contadina* Pasta Ready) 50
w/olives (*Contadina* Pasta Ready) 60
paste or puree, see "Tomato paste" and "Tomato puree"
w/red pepper, crushed (*Contadina* Pasta Ready) 60
stewed, all varieties (*Contadina*) 40
stewed, all varieties except Italian (*Del Monte*) 35
stewed, Italian (*Del Monte*) 30
wedges (*Del Monte*) 35
Tomato, dried:
(*Frieda's* No Salt), 1 oz. 86
in oil, drained (*Sonoma* Spice Medley), 1 tbsp. 50
pasta toss (*Sonoma*), ½ cup 70
Tomato, pickled:
(*Hebrew National/Shorr's*), 1 oz. 4
half sour (*Rosoff*), 1 oz. 5
Tomato, sun-dried, see "Tomato, dried"
Tomato juice, 8 fl. oz.:
(*Campbell's*) 50
(*Del Monte*) 50
(*Del Monte* Not from Concentrate) 40

Tomato paste, 2 tbsp., except as noted:

(*Del Monte*) 30

(*Progresso*) 30

Italian (*Contadina*) 40

Tomato pesto, see "Pesto sauce"

Tomato puree, regular or thick (*Progresso*), ¼ cup 25

Tomato sauce, canned (see also "Pasta sauce" and "Tomato, canned"), ¼ cup

(*Contadina/Contadina* Thick & Zesty) 20

(*Del Monte/Del Monte* No Salt) 20

(*Goya*) 20

(*Progresso*) 20

Italian (*Contadina*) 15

Tomato-beef cocktail (*Beefamato*), 8 fl. oz. 80

Tomato-clam cocktail (*Clamato*), 8 fl. oz. 100

Tongue, braised, 4 oz.:

beef 321

pork 307

veal (calf) 229

Tongue lunch meat, beef (*Hebrew National*), 2 oz. 120

Tortellini (See also "Tortelloni"), frozen or refrigerated:

cheese (*Contadina*), ¾ cup 260

cheese (*Di Giorno*), ¾ cup 260

cheese, three (*Contadina*), ¾ cup 250

chicken, herb (*Contadina*), ¾ cup 260

w/meat (*Di Giorno*), ¾ cup 290

spinach (*Contadina*), ¾ cup 270

tofu (*Soy-Boy*), ⅞ cup 190

tofu (*Tofutti*), 1 cup 320

Tortellini entree, canned, 1 cup, except as noted:

cheese (*Franco-American*) 240

meat (*Franco-American*) 260

ground beef (*Chef Boyardee*), 7½ oz. 220

Tortelloni, refrigerated, 1 cup:

cheese and basil (*Contadina*) 360

cheese and garlic (*Contadina*) 280

w/chicken and herbs (*Di Giorno*) 260

chicken and prosciutto (*Contadina*) 350

hot red pepper and cheese (*Di Giorno*) 310

mozzarella garlic (*Di Giorno*) 300

mushroom (*Contadina*) 310
mushroom (*Di Giorno*) 290
sausage (*Contadina*) 320
Tortilla, 1 piece, except as noted:
corn, white (*Goya*), 2 pieces 120
flour (*Goya*) 110
flour (*Old El Paso*) 140
flour, refrigerated (*Old El Paso*) 130
flour, refrigerated (*Old El Paso* Low Fat) 110
soft taco (*Old El Paso*), 2 pieces 170
soft taco, refrigerated (*Old El Paso*) 110
Tortilla chips, see "Corn chips, puffs, and similar
    snacks"
Tortilla mix, flour (*Burris Light Crust*), ⅓ cup 160
Tostaco or tostada shell, see "Taco shell"
Trail mix:
(*Eden* Fruit & Nuts), 1 oz. 160
California (*Dole*), 2 oz. 220
California (*Eden* Harvest), 1 oz. 130
Hawaiian (*Dole*), 2 oz. 250
Sierra (*Del Monte*), 1 oz. 120
Trout (see also "Sea trout"), meat only, 4 oz.:
mixed species, raw 168
mixed species, baked, broiled, or microwaved 215
rainbow, farmed, raw 156
rainbow, farmed, baked, broiled, or microwaved 192
rainbow, wild, raw 135
rainbow, wild, baked, broiled, or microwaved 170
Trout, smoked, peppered (*Spence & Co.*), 2 oz. 100
Tuna, meat only, 4 oz.:
bluefin, raw 163
bluefin, baked, broiled, or microwaved 209
skipjack, raw 117
skipjack, baked, broiled, or microwaved 150
yellowfin, raw 123
yellowfin, baked, broiled, or microwaved 158
Tuna, canned, drained, 2 oz. or ¼ cup:
chunk light, oil (*Bumble Bee*) 110
chunk light, oil (*Chicken of the Sea*) 110
chunk light, oil (*StarKist*) 110

Tuna, canned *(cont.)*
chunk light, water (*Bumble Bee*) 60
chunk light or white, in water (*StarKist*) 60
fillet, in water (*StarKist* Prime Light) 60
solid, olive oil (*Progresso*) 160
solid white, oil (*Bumble Bee*) 90
solid white, oil (*Chicken of the Sea*) 90
solid white, oil (*StarKist*) 90
solid white, in water (*Bumble Bee*) 70
solid white, in water (*StarKist*) 70
Tuna, frozen, yellowtail (*Peter Pan*), 4 oz. 110
Tuna casserole, frozen, noodle:
(*Stouffer's*), 10 oz. 320
(*Weight Watchers*), 9.5 oz. 270
Tuna entree mix*:
au gratin, creamy broccoli, garden cheddar, fettuccine
   Alfredo, or tetrazzini (*Tuna Helper*), 1 cup 310
pasta, creamy (*Tuna Helper*), 1 cup 300
pasta salad (*Tuna Helper*), 1 cup 380
potpie (*Tuna Helper*), 1 cup 440
Romanoff or cheesy pasta (*Tuna Helper*), 1 cup 280
Tuna spread:
(*Underwood*), ¼ cup 50
salad (*Bumble Bee*), 2.75-oz. can 70
salad, w/crackers (*Bumble Bee*), 2.75-oz. can 150
salad, w/crackers (*StarKist* Tuna Salad), 1 pkg. 190
Turbot, European, meat only, 4 oz.:
raw 108
baked, broiled, or microwaved 138
Turkey, fresh, roasted, 4 oz., except as noted:
meat w/skin 236
meat only 193
meat only, diced, 1 cup 238
skin only, 1 oz. 125
dark meat, w/skin 251
dark meat, meat only 212
dark meat, meat only, diced, 1 cup 262
light meat, w/skin 223
light meat, meat only 178
light meat, meat only, diced, 1 cup 219

back, meat w/skin 276
breast, meat w/skin, ½ breast, 1.9 lb. (4.2 lb. raw
   w/bone) 1,637
breast, meat w/skin 214
ground, see "Turkey, ground"
leg, meat w/skin, 1 leg, 1.2 lb. (1.5 lb. raw
   w/bone) 1,133
leg, meat w/skin 236
wing, meat w/skin, 1 wing, 6.6 oz. (9.9 oz. raw
   w/bone) 426
wing, meat w/skin 260
Turkey, canned, chunk, 2 oz., ¼ cup:
(*Hormel*) 70
(*Swanson* Premium) 100
white (*Hormel*) 60
white (*Swanson* Premium) 90
Turkey, frozen or refrigerated:
whole, raw, young, 4 oz.:
   (*Norbest* Family Tradition, 8–16 lb.) 190
   (*Norbest* Family Tradition, 16–24 lb.) 170
   (*Norbest,* 8–16 lb.) 180
   basted (*Norbest,* 16–24 lb.) 165
whole, cooked, dark meat (*Perdue*), 3 oz. 200
whole, cooked, white meat (*Perdue*), 3 oz. 170
whole, cooked, barbecued (*Empire* Kosher), 5 oz. 250
breast, raw, basted (*Norbest*), 4 oz. 170
breast, raw, boneless (*Perdue*), 4 oz. 130
breast, raw, cutlets, thin sliced (*Perdue*), 3½ oz. 100
breast, raw, fillets or tenderloins (*Perdue*), 4 oz. 120
breast, raw, roast, boneless (*Norbest*), 4 oz. 135
breast, cooked (*Perdue* Whole/Half), 3 oz. 170
breast, cooked, boneless, fillets or tenderloins (*Perdue*),
   3 oz. 110
breast, cooked, cutlets, thin sliced (*Perdue*), 2.5 oz. 90
breast, oven roasted (*Hebrew National*), 2 oz. 60
breast, oven-roasted, skinless (*Hebrew National*), 2 oz. . . 50
breast, smoked (*Hebrew National*), 2 oz. 60
breast, smoked (*Hormel Light & Lean* 97), 3 oz. 80
breast, smoked (*Perdue*), 3 oz. 150
ground, see "Turkey, ground"

Turkey, frozen or refrigerated *(cont.)*

maple glaze (*Boar's Head Honey Coat*), 3 oz. 100
roast, boneless (*Norbest*), 4 oz. 135
smoked, hickory (*Norbest* Young), 3 oz. 145
steak, cubed, raw (*Perdue*), 4 oz. 110
thigh, cooked (*Perdue*), 3 oz. 180
wing, cooked (*Perdue* Tom), 3 oz. 160
wing, cooked, portion (*Perdue*), 3 oz. 170
wing, roasted (*Perdue*), 3-oz. wing 180
wing, roasted (*Perdue* Drummettes), 3½-oz. piece 180

Turkey, ground:

raw (*Norbest*), 4 oz. 170
raw (*Shady Brook Farms*), 4 oz. 170
raw, breast (*Shady Brook Farms*), 4 oz. 120
cooked, breast (*Perdue*), 3 oz. 110
cooked, regular or burger (*Perdue*), 3 oz. 170

"Turkey," vegetarian:

canned (*Worthington* Turkee), 3 slices 190
frozen, smoked (*Worthington*), 3 slices 140

Turkey bacon (*Louis Rich*), .5-oz. slice 30
Turkey bologna (*Empire*), 3 slices 90
Turkey dinner, frozen, 1 pkg.:

breast (*Healthy Choice*), 10.5 oz. 280
breast, stuffed (*The Budget Gourmet*), 11 oz. 240
and gravy, w/dressing (*Freezer Queen* Meal), 9.2 oz. . . . 210
and gravy, w/dressing (*Marie Callender's*), 14 oz. 530
roast (*Healthy Choice* Country Inn), 10 oz. 250

Turkey entree, canned:

gravy and dressing (*Libby's Diner*), 7 oz. 180
stew (*Dinty Moore* Cup), 7.5 oz. 130

Turkey entree, frozen, 1 pkg., except as noted:

(*Lean Cuisine* Homestyle), 9⅜ oz. 240
breast, stuffed (*Weight Watchers*), 9 oz. 230
croquettes, gravy and (*Freezer Queen* Family), 1 patty
     and gravy, 4.65 oz. 130
glazed (*The Budget Gourmet* Light), 9 oz. 250
and gravy, w/dressing (*Freezer Queen* Deluxe Family),
     ¼ of 28-oz. pkg. 170
and gravy, w/dressing (*Freezer Queen* Homestyle),
     9 oz. 210

gravy and (*Freezer Queen* Family), 4.5 oz. 60
medallions (*Smart Ones*), 8.5 oz. 190
pie (*Lean Cuisine*), 9.5 oz. 320
pie (*Marie Callender's*), 1 cup, 8.5 oz. 740
pie (*Stouffer's*), 10-oz. pie 530
pie (*Tyson*), 8.9 oz. 470
roast, breast, and stuffing (*Lean Cuisine*), 9¾ oz. 290
roast, w/mushrooms (*Healthy Choice* Country),
    8.5 oz. 220
roast, and stuffing (*Stouffer's* Homestyle), 9⅝ oz. 320
sliced, gravy and (*Freezer Queen* Cook-in-Pouch), 5 oz. . . 70
and vegetables (*Healthy Choice Hearty Handfuls*), 6.1 oz. 310
Turkey entree, refrigerated:
nuggets, breaded (*Louis Rich*), 4 pieces 260
patty, breaded (*Louis Rich*), 3-oz. piece 220
sticks, breaded (*Louis Rich*), 3 pieces 230
Turkey frankfurter, 1 link:
and beef (*Oscar Mayer* Fat Free) 40
and chicken (*Louis Rich* 8 links/12 oz.), 1.5 oz. 80
Turkey giblets, simmered, chopped or diced, 1 cup . . . 243
Turkey gravy, ¼ cup:
(*Heinz* Home Style) 30
seasoned, w/turkey (*Pepperidge Farm*) 30
mix* (*McCormick*) 20
Turkey ham:
(*Louis Rich* Chunk), 2 oz. 70
(*Louis Rich*), 1-oz. slice 30
(*Louis Rich Deli-Thin*), 4 slices, 2 oz. 60
canned (*Hormel*), 2 oz. 70
chopped (*Louis Rich*), 1-oz. slice 40
Turkey lunch meat (see also "Turkey ham," etc.), breast,
    2 oz., except as noted:
(*Boar's Head* Premium Lower Sodium/Premium Lower
    Sodium Skinless) 60
(*Hormel* Deli Premium/*Hormel Light & Lean 97*) 50
honey roasted (*Louis Rich*) 60
maple honey (*Boar's Head*) 70
oven roasted (*Boar's Head* Golden/Golden Skinless) 60
oven roasted (*Hebrew National*), 5 thin slices 50
oven roasted (*Louis Rich*) 50

Turkey lunch meat *(cont.)*
oven roasted (*Oscar Mayer*), 1-oz. slice 30
rotisserie flavor (*Louis Rich*) 50
rotisserie flavor (*Louis Rich Carving Board*), 2 slices 45
skinless (*Hormel/Hormel* Deli) 50
smoked (*Boar's Head* Hickory) 70
smoked (*Empire*), 3 slices 40
smoked (*Hebrew National* Hickory) 60
smoked (*Hormel* Mesquite) 60
smoked (*Hormel Light & Lean* 97 Mesquite), 1 oz. 30
smoked (*Louis Rich* Hickory) 50
smoked (*Louis Rich Carving Board*), 2 slices 40
Turkey nuggets, breaded (*Louis Rich*), 4 pieces, 3.25 oz. 260
Turkey pastrami:
(*Empire*), 3 slices 60
(*Hebrew National*), 2 oz. 60
(*Louis Rich* Chunk), 2 oz. 60
Turkey patty, breaded (*Empire* Kosher), 1 piece 200
Turkey pie, see "Turkey entree"
Turkey salami:
(*Empire*), 3 slices 70
(*Louis Rich* Chunk), 2 oz. 120
cotto (*Louis Rich*), 1-oz. slice 40
Turkey sandwich, frozen, 4.5-oz. piece:
w/broccoli and cheese (*Lean Pockets*) 260
and ham w/cheese (*Hot Pockets*) 320
and ham w/cheese (*Lean Pockets*) 270
and ham w/Swiss (*Croissant Pockets*) 300
Turkey sausage, raw, except as noted:
breakfast, raw (*Shady Brook Farms*), 4 oz. 160
Italian, hot or sweet (*Louis Rich*), 2.5 oz. 120
Italian, hot or sweet (*Shady Brook Farms*), 4 oz. 170
smoked (*Louis Rich/Louis Rich* Polska), 2 oz. 90
smoked, and duck, cooked (*Gerhard's*), 2.5 oz. 100
Turkey seasoning, w/gravy (*McCormick Bag 'n Season*),
  1 tsp. 15
Turkey spread:
chunky (*Underwood*), ¼ cup 110
salad (*Libby's Spreadables*), ⅓ cup 150
Turkey sticks, breaded (*Louis Rich*), 3 pieces 230

Turnip:

fresh or stored, boiled, drained, mashed, ½ cup 21

frozen, boiled, drained, 4 oz. 26

Turnip greens, ½ cup:

fresh, raw, chopped 7

fresh, boiled, drained, chopped 15

canned (*Stubb's Harvest*) 25

frozen, w/diced turnips (*Seabrook*) 30

Turnover, frozen, 1 piece, except as noted:

apple (*Pillsbury*), 2 pieces 350

apple or raspberry (*Pepperidge Farm*) 330

blueberry or peach (*Pepperidge Farm*) 340

cherry (*Pepperidge Farm*) 320

cherry (*Pillsbury*), 2 pieces 360

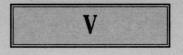

FOOD AND MEASURE

CALORIES

Veal, meat only, 4 oz.:
cubed, lean only, braised or stewed 213
ground, broiled 195
leg, braised, lean w/fat 239
leg, braised, lean only 230
leg, roasted, lean w/fat 181
leg, roasted, lean only 170
loin, braised, lean w/fat 322
loin, braised, lean only 256
loin, roasted, lean w/fat 246
loin, roasted, lean only 198
rib, roasted, lean w/fat 259
rib, roasted, lean only 201
shoulder, whole, braised, lean w/fat 259
shoulder, whole, braised, lean only 226
shoulder, whole, roasted, lean w/fat 209
shoulder, whole, roasted, lean only 193
shoulder, arm, braised, lean w/fat 268
shoulder, arm, braised, lean only 228
shoulder, blade, braised, lean w/fat 255
shoulder, blade, braised, lean only 224
sirloin, braised, lean w/fat 286
sirloin, braised, lean only 231
sirloin, roasted, lean w/fat 229
sirloin, roasted, lean only 191
Veal dinner, parmigiana, frozen (*Freezer Queen* Meal),
 10.2 oz. 290
Veal entree, parmigiana, frozen:
(*Banquet*), 9 oz. 320
(*Freezer Queen* Deluxe Family), 4.9-oz. patty 170
breaded, w/tomato sauce (*Freezer Queen* Cook-in-Pouch),
 5 oz. 190
w/spaghetti (*Stouffer's* Homestyle), 11^{7}/$_{8}$ oz. 430

patties (*Banquet* Family), 4.7-oz. patty 230
Vegetable burger, see " 'Hamburger,' vegetarian"
Vegetable chips:
(*Eden*), 50 chips, 1.1 oz. 130
sea (*Eden*), 50 chips, 1.1 oz. 140
Vegetable entree, frozen, 1 pkg., except as noted:
Chinese, and chicken (*The Budget Gourmet* Special
    Selections), 9 oz. 260
country, and beef (*Lean Cuisine*), 9 oz. 220
Italian, and chicken (*The Budget Gourmet* Special
    Selections), 9 oz. 240
pie (*Amy's*), 7.5 oz. 360
pie (*Amy's* Nondairy), 7.5 oz. 320
pie, broccoli and cheese (*Tyson*), 8.9-oz. pie 210
pie, w/cheese (*Banquet*), 7-oz. pie 390
pie, shepherd's, nondairy (*Amy's*), 8-oz. pie 160
Szechuan style, and chicken (*The Budget Gourmet*
    Special Selections), 10 oz. 330
Vegetable juice, 8 fl. oz.:
(*V-8* Plus 100%) 50
original, picante or spicy hot (*V-8* 100%) 50
tangy (*V-8* 100%) 60
Vegetable oyster, see "Salsify"
Vegetable pie, see "Vegetable entree"
Vegetable pocket (see also specific listings), frozen,
    1 piece:
Bar-B-Q (*Ken & Robert's Veggie Pockets*) 290
Greek or Oriental (*Ken & Robert's Veggie Pockets*) . . . 250
Indian (*Ken & Robert's Veggie Pockets*) 260
pizza (*Ken & Robert's Veggie Pockets*) 270
potpie (*Amy's Pocketfuls*) 230
potpie (*Ken & Robert's Veggie Pockets*) 250
Santa Fe (*Ken & Robert's Veggie Pockets*) 250
Tex-Mex (*Ken & Robert's Veggie Pockets*) 280
Vegetables, see specific listings
Vegetables, mixed:
fresh, California, garden, or Oriental style (*Dole*), 3 oz. . . 30
fresh, Italian style (*Dole*), 3 oz. 25
fresh, New England (*Dole*), 3 oz. 50
canned (*Del Monte/Del Monte* No Salt), ½ cup 40

Vegetables, mixed *(cont.)*

canned (*Goya*), ½ cup	35
canned (*Green Giant*), ½ cup	60
canned (*Green Giant Garden Medley*), ½ cup	40
canned (*Seneca/Seneca* No Salt), ½ cup	45
canned, stew (*Seneca*), ½ cup	45
frozen (*Goya*), ⅔ cup	60
frozen (*Green Giant*), ¾ cup	50
frozen, butter sauce (*Green Giant*), ¾ cup	70
frozen, soup (*Birds Eye*), ⅔ cup	45
frozen, stew (*Ore-Ida*), ⅔ cup	50
frozen, stir-fry (*Birds Eye*), 1 cup	30
frozen, tropical (*Goya* Pasteles de Masa), 1 pkg.	280
frozen, tropical (*Goya* Viando Sancocho), 3 oz.	100
frozen, tropical (*Goya* Yautia Malanga), ⅛ pkg.	130

Vegetables, mixed, pickled (*Krinos*), 3 oz. 0
Vegetarian burger, see " 'Hamburger,' vegetarian"
Vegetarian entree (see also specific listings):

canned (*Loma Linda Swiss Stake*), 1 piece	120
canned (*Worthington Numete*), ⅜" slice	130
canned (*Worthington Protose*), ⅜" slice	130
canned, choplet (*Worthington*), 2 pieces	90
canned cuts, dinner (*Loma Linda*), 2 pieces	90
canned, cutlet (*Worthington*), 1 piece	70
frozen (*Worthington FriPats*), 1 patty	130
frozen (*Worthington Stakelets*), 1 piece	140
frozen, croquettes (*Worthington* Golden), 4 pieces	210
frozen, dinner entree (*Natural Touch*), 3-oz. patty	220
frozen, nuggets, w/rice (*Hain* Hawaiian), 10 oz.	310
frozen, roast, dinner (*Worthington*), ¾" slice	180
mix, dry (*Loma Linda* Dinner Loaf/Patty), ⅓ cup	90

Venison, meat only, roasted, 4 oz. 179
Vienna sausage, canned:

(*Goya*), 4 links	170
(*Hormel*), 2 oz.	140
(*Libby's/Libby's* BBQ), 3 links	130
w/hot sauce (*Goya*), 3 links	130
chicken (*Hormel*), 2 oz.	110
chicken (*Libby's*), 3 links	100

Vine spinach, raw, untrimmed, 1 lb. 86
Vinegar, 1 tbsp.:
all varieties (*Progresso*) 0
balsamic (*Pastorelli Italian Chef*) 5
red wine (*Pastorelli Italian Chef*) 2

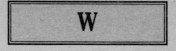

W

FOOD AND MEASURE	CALORIES

Waffle, frozen, 2 pieces, except as noted:
(*Belgian Chef*), 1 piece 170
(*Eggo* Homestyle) 220
(*Nutri-Grain*) 190
apple cinnamon, blueberry, buttermilk, or strawberry
    (*Eggo*) 220
blueberry (*Aunt Jemima*) 190
buttermilk (*Aunt Jemima*) 170
cinnamon (*Aunt Jemima*) 180
multibran (*Nutri-Grain*) 80
nut and honey (*Eggo*) 240
oat bran (*Common Sense*) 200
oat bran, w/fruit and nut (*Common Sense*) 220
oatmeal or whole grain (*Aunt Jemima*) 170
raisin and bran (*Nutri-Grain*) 210
Waffle mix, see "Pancake mix"
Walnut, dried:
(*Paradise/Wild Swan*), ¼ cup, 1 oz. 190
black (*Planters*), 2-oz. pkg. 340
black, chopped, 1 cup 759
English or Persian, pieces, 1 cup 770
halves (*Planters Gold Measure*), 2-oz. pkg. 380
pieces (*Planters*), ¼ cup 190
Walnut topping, in syrup (*Smucker's*), 2 tbsp. 190
Wasabi chips (*Eden*), 50 pieces, 1.1 oz. 130
Water chestnuts, canned (*La Choy*), 2 whole 10
Watercress, fresh, chopped, ½ cup 2
Watermelon:
(*Dole*), 1/18 medium melon, 10 oz. 90
seedless (*Frieda's*), 1 oz. 7
Watermelon drink (*Hi-C Watermelon Rapids*), 8.45 oz. ... 120
Watermelon rind, sweet (*Haddon House*), 2 cubes,
    1 oz. 70

Watermelon seed, dried, 1 oz. 158
Wax beans:
canned, cut (*Seneca/Seneca* No Salt), ½ cup 25
canned, golden, cut (*Del Monte*), ½ cup 20
frozen (*Seabrook*), ⅔ cup 25
Welsh rarebit, frozen (*Stouffer's*), 2.2 oz. 120
Wendy's, 1 serving:
sandwiches:
   bacon cheeseburger, Jr. 380
   Big Bacon Classic 570
   cheeseburger, Jr. or Kid's Meal 320
   cheeseburger deluxe, Jr. 360
   chicken, grilled 310
   chicken, breaded 440
   chicken, spicy 410
   chicken club 470
   hamburger, single, plain 360
   hamburger, single, w/everything 420
   hamburger, Jr. or Kid's Meal 270
sandwich components:
   American cheese 70
   American cheese, Jr. 45
   bacon, 1 slice 20
   bun, kaiser 190
   bun, sandwich 160
   burger patty, ¼ lb. 200
   burger patty, 2 oz. 100
   chicken patty, grilled 110
   chicken patty, breaded 230
   chicken patty, spicy 210
   honey mustard, reduced calorie, 1 tsp. 25
   ketchup, 1 tsp. 10
   lettuce, 1 leaf 0
   mayonnaise, 1½ tsp. 30
   mustard, ½ tsp. 0
   onion or pickles, 4 rings or slices 0
   tomato, 1 slice 5
chicken nuggets, 5 pieces 210
nuggets sauces, 1 oz.:
   barbecue or sweet and sour 50

Wendy's, nuggets sauces *(cont.)*

 honey mustard 130
 spicy buffalo wing 25

chili:

 small, 8 oz. 210
 large, 12 oz. 340
 cheddar cheese, shredded, 2 tbsp. 70
 Saltines crackers, 2 pieces 25

baked potato:

 plain 310
 bacon and cheese 540
 broccoli and cheese 470
 cheese 570
 chili and cheese 620
 sour cream and chive 380
 sour cream or whipped margarine, 1 pkt. 60

breadstick, soft, 1 piece 130

fries:

 small, 3.2 oz. 260
 medium, 4.6 oz. 380
 Biggie, 5.6 oz. 460

salads-to-go, fresh, w/out dressing:

 deluxe garden 110
 grilled chicken 200
 grilled chicken Caesar 260
 side salad 60
 side salad, Caesar 110
 taco salad 590

salad dressing, 2 tbsp., except as noted:

 blue cheese 170
 French 120
 French, fat free 30
 French, sweet red 130
 Italian, reduced fat and calorie 40
 Italian Caesar 150
 ranch, *Hidden Valley* 90
 ranch, *Hidden Valley,* reduced fat and calorie 60
 salad oil, 1 tbsp. 130
 Thousand Island 130
 wine vinegar, 1 tbsp. 0

Garden Spot salad bar:

applesauce, 2 tbsp. 30
bacon bits, 2 tbsp. 45
banana & strawberry glaze, ¼ cup 30
broccoli or cauliflower, ¼ cup 0
cantaloupe, 1 slice 15
cheese, shredded, imitation, 2 tbsp. 50
chicken salad, 2 tbsp. 70
chow mein noodles, ¼ cup 35
coleslaw, 2 tbsp. 45
cottage cheese, 2 tbsp. 30
croutons, 2 tbsp. 30
cucumbers, 2 slices 0
eggs, hard-cooked, 2 tbsp. 40
green peas, 2 tbsp. 15
green pepper, 2 pieces 0
honeydew, 1 slice 20
lettuce, 1 cup 10
mushrooms, ½ cup 0
orange, 2 slices 15
Parmesan blend, grated, 2 tbsp. 70
pasta salad, 2 tbsp. 25
peaches, 1 slice 15
pepperoni, 6 slices 30
pineapple chunks, 4 pieces 20
potato salad, 2 tbsp. 80
pudding, chocolate or vanilla, ¼ cup 70
red onion, 3 rings 0
seafood salad, ¼ cup 70
sesame breadstick, 1 piece 15
strawberries, 1 piece 10
sunflower seeds and raisins, 2 tbsp. 80
tomato wedges, 1 piece 5
turkey ham, diced, 2 tbsp. 50
watermelon, 1 wedge 20
desserts:

chocolate chip cookie, 1 piece 270
Frosty, small 340
Frosty, medium 460
Frosty, large 570

Western entree, frozen (*Banquet* Country), 9.5 oz. 350
Wheat, whole grain:
durum, 1 cup 650
hard red, winter (*Arrowhead Mills*), ¼ cup 160
soft red, winter, 1 cup 556
hard white, 1 cup 656
soft white, 1 cup 571
Wheat, parboiled, see "Bulgur"
Wheat, sprouted, 1 cup 214
Wheat bran (see also "Cereal")
(*Shiloh Farms*), ¼ cup 30
toasted (*Kretschmer*), ¼ cup 30
unprocessed (*Quaker*), ⅓ cup 30
Wheat flakes (*Arrowhead Mills*), ⅓ cup 110
Wheat flour, ¼ cup, except as noted:
(*Wondra*) 100
all-purpose, white:
    (*Gold Medal*) 100
    unbleached (*Arrowhead Mills*), ⅓ cup 160
    unbleached (*Gold Medal*) 100
    unbleached, whole grain (*Arrowhead Mills*) 110
cake, white (*Betty Crocker Softasilk*) 100
bread, wheat blend (*Gold Medal*) 110
bread, white (*Gold Medal*) 100
gluten (*Arrowhead Mills*), 3 tbsp. 35
gluten (*General Mills* Supreme Hygluten) 100
HD (*Gladiola*) 120
pastry, soft, white, unbleached (*Arrowhead Mills*) 100
pastry, soft, whole grain (*Arrowhead Mills*), ⅓ cup 100
self-rising, white (*Gold Medal*) 100
whole grain, stone ground (*Arrowhead Mills*) 130
whole wheat (*Gold Medal*) 90
Wheat germ:
(*Kretschmer*), 2 tbsp. 50
honey crunch (*Kretschmer*), 1⅔ tbsp. 50
raw (*Arrowhead Mills*), 3 tbsp. 50
Wheat nuts (*Sonoma*), 2 tbsp. 60
Wheat pilaf mix (*Near East*), 1 cup* 220
Whelk, meat only, raw, 4 oz. 156
Whipped topping, see "Cream topping"

Whiskey sour mixer:
bottled (*Holland House*), 4 fl. oz. 150
bottled (*Mr & Mrs T*), 4 fl. oz. 100
mix (*Bar-Tenders*), 2 pkts. 130
mix (*Bar-Tenders* Lite), 3 pkts. 20
mix (*Bar-Tenders* Slightly Sour), 2 pkts. 120
White bean, ½ cup:
dried, boiled 125
canned (*Goya*) 80
canned, in tomato sauce (*Goya* Guisados) 110
White sauce mix (*Knorr*), ⅛ pkg. 25
Whitefish, meat only, 4 oz.:
raw 153
baked, broiled, or microwaved 195
smoked 122
Whiting, meat only, 4 oz.:
raw 102
baked, broiled, or microwaved 130
Wiener, see "Frankfurter"
Wild rice:
raw (*Fantastic Foods*), ¼ cup 140
cooked, 1 cup 166
blends, see "Rice"
Wild rice dishes, see "Rice dishes"
Wine, 1 fl. oz.:
dessert or aperitif (sherry, port, vermouth, etc.) 41
dry or table (burgundy, Chablis, champagne, rosé, etc.) . . 25
Wine, cooking, 2 tbsp.:
(*La Viña* Gold/Red/White) 2
all varieties except Marsala and sherry (*Holland House*) . . 20
Marsala (*Holland House*) 35
sherry (*Holland House*) 45
Winged beans, ½ cup:
fresh, boiled, drained 12
dried, boiled 126
Winged bean leaves, trimmed, 1 oz. 21
Winged bean tuber, trimmed, 1 oz. 45
Wolffish, Atlantic, meat only, 4 oz.:
raw 109
baked, broiled, or microwaved 139

Wonton wrapper (*Frieda's*), 4 pieces 80
Worcestershire sauce, 1 tsp.:
(*French's*) 0
(*Lea & Perrins*) 5
white wine (*Lea & Perrins*) 0

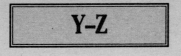

Y–Z

FOOD AND MEASURE   **CALORIES**

Yam:
baked or boiled, ½ cup 79
canned or frozen, see "Sweet potato"
Yam, mountain, Hawaiian, steamed, cubed, ½ cup 59
Yam bean tuber, raw (*Frieda's*), 3.5 oz. 45
Yard-long bean, ½ cup:
fresh, sliced, raw 22
dried, raw 292
Yeast, baker's, all varieties (*Fleischmann's*), ¼ tsp. 0
Yellow bean, dried, boiled, ½ cup 126
Yellow squash:
fresh or frozen, see "Crookneck squash"
canned (*Allens/Sunshine*), ½ cup 25
Yellowtail, meat only, 4 oz.:
raw 166
baked, broiled, or microwaved 212
Yogurt, 1 cup or 8 oz., except as noted:
plain (*Breyers*) 130
plain (*Friendship*) 150
all flavors (*Colombo* Light) 100
all flavors (*Dannon* Light) 100
all flavors (*Weight Watchers* Nonfat) 90
all flavors (*Yoplait* Custard Style), 6 oz. 190
all flavors, except banana creme strawberry (*Dannon*
  Double Delights) 170
all fruit flavors (*Dannon* Fruit on Bottom) 240
all fruit flavors (*Light n'Lively Free* 50 Cal), 4.4 oz. 50
all fruit flavors, except banana/strawberry (*Colombo* Fat
  Free) 200
banana (*Tropifruita*), 6 oz. 150
banana creme strawberry (*Dannon Double Delights*),
  6 oz. 160
banana/strawberry (*Colombo* Fat Free) 220

Yogurt *(cont.)*

berry, mixed (*Breyers*) 250
berry, mixed (*Light n'Lively Free*), 6 oz. 170
blueberry (*Breyers*) 250
blueberry (*Light n'Lively Free*), 6 oz. 190
blueberry and creme (*Ultimate 90*) 90
cappuccino (*Ultimate 90*) 90
cappuccino, all flavors (*Colombo* Fat Free) 170
cherry, black (*Breyers*) 260
cherry jubilee (*Ultimate 90*) 90
coffee (*Breyers*) 220
cranberry raspberry (*Ultimate 90*) 90
guava (*Tropifruita*), 6 oz. 150
lemon (*Light n'Lively Free*), 6 oz. 170
lemon, creamy (*Breyers*) 220
lemon chiffon (*Ultimate 90*) 90
mango (*Tropifruita*), 6 oz. 150
papaya-pineapple (*Tropifruita*), 6 oz. 150
peach (*Breyers*) 250
peach (*Light n'Lively Free*), 6 oz. 170
peach (*Ultimate 90*) 90
piña colada (*Tropifruita*), 6 oz. 150
pineapple (*Breyers*) 250
raspberry creme (*Ultimate 90*) 90
raspberry or strawberry (*Breyers*) 250
raspberry or strawberry (*Light n'Lively Free*), 6 oz. . . 180
strawberry (*Tropifruita*), 6 oz. 150
strawberry (*Ultimate 90*) 90
strawberry, fruit cup (*Light n'Lively Free*), 6 oz. . . . 170
strawberry-banana (*Breyers*) 250
strawberry-banana (*Tropifruita*), 6 oz. 150
strawberry-banana (*Ultimate 90*) 90
strawberry-kiwi (*Tropifruita*), 6 oz. 150
vanilla (*Breyers*) 220
vanilla (*Light n'Lively Free*), 6 oz. 160
vanilla (*Ultimate 90*) 90
Yogurt, frozen, ½ cup, except as noted:
all flavors (*Colombo* Cooler) 60
all flavors (*Dannon* Fat Free Soft) 100
all flavors (*Dannon* Light 'n Crunchy) 110

all flavors except caramel praline crunch, cookies in
   cream, and vanilla fudge twirl (*Breyers* Fat Free) . . . 100
all flavors except peanut butter (*Colombo* Lowfat) 110
banana pudding, homestyle (*TCBY*) 120
butter pecan (*Breyers*) 170
cappuccino (*Ben & Jerry's* No Fat) 140
caramel praline crunch (*Breyers* Fat Free) 120
caramel praline crunch (*Edy's/Dreyer's* Fat Free) 100
cherry, black, vanilla swirl (*Edy's/Dreyer's* Fat Free) 80
cherry chocolate chunk (*Edy's/Dreyer's*) 110
chocolate (*Breyers*) 130
chocolate (*Dannon* Lowfat Soft) 120
chocolate brownie chunk (*Edy's/Dreyer's*) 120
chocolate chip cookie dough (*Breyers*) 150
chocolate chip cup (*Breyers*), 1 piece 230
chocolate chip mint (*Breyers*) 140
chocolate fudge (*Edy's/Dreyer's* Fat Free) 100
chocolate silk mousse (*Edy's/Dreyer's* Fat Free) 90
coffee fudge (*Ben & Jerry's* No Fat) 140
coffee fudge sundae (*Edy's/Dreyer's* Fat Free) 100
cone crunch, crispy (*TCBY*) 130
cookies and cream (*Breyers* Fat Free) 110
cookies and cream (*Edy's/Dreyer's*) 120
cookies and cream (*TCBY*) 120
cookie dough (*Edy's/Dreyer's*) 130
marble fudge (*Edy's/Dreyer's* Fat Free) 100
peach (*Breyers*) 120
peach (*TCBY*) 110
peanut butter (*Colombo* Lowfat) 120
peanut butter (*Dannon* Lowfat Soft) 120
peanut butter fudge sundae (*TCBY*) 110
pecan praline crisp (*TCBY*) 110
raspberry, black, swirl (*Ben & Jerry's* No Fat) 150
raspberry sorbet 'n cream (*Edy's/Dreyer's* Fat Free) 90
(*Starburst*), 1 cup 80
strawberry (*Breyers*) 120
strawberry, summertime (*TCBY*) 100
strawberry cheesecake (*Breyers*) 130
toffee crunch (*Edy's/Dreyer's* Heath) 120
toffee crunch bar (*Breyers*) 140

Yogurt, frozen *(cont.)*
vanilla (*Breyers*) 130
vanilla (*Dannon* Lowfat Soft) 110
vanilla (*Edy's/Dreyer's*) 100
vanilla (*Edy's/Dreyer's* Fat Free) 80
vanilla, classic (*TCBY*) 110
vanilla, French (*Breyers*) 110
vanilla chocolate swirl (*Edy's/Dreyer's* Fat Free) 80
vanilla-chocolate-strawberry combination (*Breyers*) 120
vanilla fudge swirl (*Ben & Jerry's* No Fat) 140
vanilla fudge twirl (*Breyers*) 130
vanilla fudge twirl (*Breyers* Fat Free) 110
vanilla raspberry truffle (*Dannon Pure Indulgence*) 150
Yogurt bar, frozen, 1 bar:
(*Creamsicle*) 60
all flavors (*Starburst*) 70
Cherry Garcia (*Ben & Jerry's* Peace Pop) 260
chocolate almond (*Frozfruit*) 130
peach, strawberry, or strawberry-banana (*Frozfruit*) 100
Yuca:
boiled, drained (*Frieda's*), 4 oz. 77
frozen (*Goya*), ½ cup 191
Ziti entree, frozen:
(*The Budget Gourmet* Value Classics), 9 oz. 350
mozzarella (*Weight Watchers*), 9 oz. 280
Zucchini:
fresh, raw, sliced, ½ cup 9
fresh, boiled, drained, sliced, ½ cup 14
canned, Italian style (*Progresso*), ½ cup 40
frozen, sliced (*Stilwell*), ⅔ cup 15
Zucchini, breaded, frozen (*Empire*), 1 piece 100
Zucchini, sun-dried, in olive oil and balsamic vinegar
(*Antica Italia*), 1 oz. 160